Becoming Whole

Building Natural Immunity
in the
Body and Soul

Second Edition

Dr. Lea Povozhaev

COPYRIGHT DISCLAIMER

Becoming Whole:
Building Natural Immunity in the Body and Soul
Paperback
1st Edition: March 2016
2nd Edition: February 2018
Alpha Academic Press
ISBN-13: 978-0-9967715-4-2
ISBN-10: 09967715-4-9
BISAC: HEA050000 – Health & Fitness/Vaccinations

Photo Credits:
Front Cover: Greek Orthodox icon of our Lord and Savior Jesus Christ "The Life- Giver"
https://www.orthodoxmonasteryicons.com/products/jesus-christ-the-life-giver-icon
Back Cover: Photo is duplicated with permission from an Orthodox Christian participant on the West Coast in the March for Life in Washington D.C., Jan. 19, 2018.

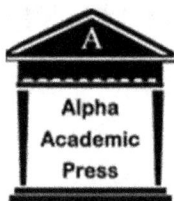

Alpha
Academic
Press

Published in the United States of America

Table of Contents

Table of Contents

ACKNOWLEDGEMENTS

Dear Dima, your quest for truth and your love for our family is the backbone of this book. My life is yours. May all children grow healthy, strong, and aware of the Giver of Life. When I first began to wonder at my crazy Russian husband's concerns over vaccination, Sister Melanie Ann Sherman, I had thought that you and Mom were too American to go there. I had wrongly worried that you wouldn't reconsider what our culture has trained us to believe. Yours and our Mom's open-minds continue a renewing gift. Your encouragement is ever-ready. Thank you, Diane and Don Patton (Mom and Dad) for sharing coffee and listening as I learned about the ills of vaccination and stumbled about trying to demystify natural immunity of the body and soul.

It has stung to face opposition to the message in this work, but, as dear Science Major friends once said: "We are helping you make this book better." What love that even though you didn't agree with me, you were willing to engage with me in heated discussions, to read countless materials I emailed to you, and to even accept *Dissolving Illusions*, by Suzanne Humphries, M.D., which I determinedly stuffed into your arms as you passed me on the way to the chalice for the Eucharist. May God draw us together in Truth and Love, my two very beloved friends. And others who have less lovingly argued with me, online groups where challenges were waged with faceless aggression: thank you. Each challenge allowed me to double-check, refine my articulation, and realize more clearly what I have to say. To family and friends Up North who do not agree: I pray you will. I love you. Thank you for your patience with my passion. Those in the Orthodox Church who turned from my message and dismissed it, this was the hardest. But I thank you for your doubt and your challenge to me as a mere child who shouldn't speak for the Church. I know what I know, and I believe what I believe, merely as a faithful Orthodox Christian. Not a priest, not a theologian, not a cradle Orthodox. A mother, a convert, and one deeply concerned with Truth—which is preserved within Orthodoxy, whose Holy Tradition I seek to understand with my life. Thank you to the priests, theologians, and skeptics within the Church who checked my passion and humbled me.

Writing this book was an "opened window" and a "closed door," and I thank the Lord: Father, Son, and Holy Spirit, for guiding me in the direction that I can now see was my road. An appreciation for St. Alexis Toth, who is a Truth-seeker and one tenderly connected to my fifth pregnancy, grows with me. "Oh Lord, save your people and bless your inheritance." St. Seraphim of Sarov, your humility and acquiescence reminds the world of being in Christ. Your words: "Acquire a peaceful spirit and thousands around you will be saved," speak a truth I aim to embrace, despite my failure to do so. And, lastly, Theotokos, many nights up with prayers to you, begging for your intercession to help and protect. The night after first meeting with Dr. Tenpenny and beginning to change my position on vaccination was riddled with fear and self-doubt, until my heart turned to you. I prayed and you were near. Thank you, mother of our God.

I became more brazen realizing that many others: doctors, scientists, and parents and concerned citizens are learning, acting, speaking out in their communities. I am grateful for the freedoms we enjoy in current America to learn, share our thoughts, and express our understandings. May this freedom remain, and may the truth spread among us concerning holistic health and authentic wellness. Thank you to individuals on the front-lines who are battling against mandatory vaccination and admitting that they stand: anti-vaccine. No splicing their words, no perpetuation of confusion, just the open and clear truth we so desperately need to set us freer. A hearty dose of gratitude for those who agreed to writing an endorsement for *Becoming Whole*, even in early stages of the manuscript's development (and for others who read and commented on the drafts): Dr. Robert Rowen, Fr. Alexis Baldwin, Barbara Feick Gregory, and Cynthia Damaskos. Each of you offers a special insight to what is included here and increases my faith in those who care for the body and soul. May God shine His light on your paths.

Daniel Stanley and Alpha Academic Press, thank you for publishing my work and for sharing in my vision for *Becoming Whole: Building Natural Immunity in the Body and Soul*. As you said, and I second, my goal is to teach others what I have found through my research and dedication. May this book carry the prayer: "Thy will be done." Thank you, readers, for taking the time and giving this thought....

Thank God for leaders in the Church who have listened and blessed my work. Fr. Alexis Baldwin, rector of Holy Resurrection Orthodox Mission in North Augusta, SC, as well as Gerondissa Michaila from St. Paisius Monastery in AZ, your prayers are much appreciated and your understanding of the severity of this issue encourages me to communicate to the Church this "much needed message." Additionally, Dcn. Stephen Muse from Holy Transfiguration Greek Orthodox Church in Columbus, GA, our friendship and communications on this topic have strengthened this message. Cynthia Damaskos, thank you for helping me speak to the Church through our podcast on Holistic Christian Life, and for sharing this book with the Orthodox Speakers Bureau.

A very sincere thank you to the Right Reverend Paul Gassios, Bishop of Chicago and the Midwest, for taking the time to read and discuss my work and blessing me to share the message I have with the Orthodox Church. Father Andrew Clements, your guidance the past 13 years since baptizing me and my growing family blesses me beyond words. Thank you for listening to this hard message and considering its need in light of current society.

FOREWORD

By *Dr. Robert Jay Rowen, MD*

The issue of religion and vaccination does not begin and end with a decision of a church leader. It begins and ends with you. I am not a "Christian" in the commonly understood meaning of the term. However, I am familiar enough with the teachings of Jesus to know that, according to him, the Kingdom of God is *within*, and does not reside in any church or church representative. There are as many ways to see God, as there are people on the planet, since none of us occupy the shoes of the other.

I respect the views of those who consider abortion as immoral. They are certainly so entitled to their views as it applies them and their families. In my opinion, they should not be forced, virtually at gunpoint, to partake of the "profits" or "benefits" of that enterprise against their will (as in forced vaccination with potions derived from aborted fetal tissue).

I have a copy of Webster's 1828 dictionary that clearly defines words used by people of his time, which was the founding period of the nation. Religion is defined as "obedience" to the Creator, "piety to God," "a system of moral beliefs and practices." It was not defined as a practice laid out by a self-proclaimed "man of God" (priest, minister, rabbi, etc.) but includes any form of obedience to a Higher Power by any so-called "religion."

As a secular, but very spiritual man, I see freedom of religion as your right to obey and serve God in your own interpretation of His commands, provided your actions do not tread on the rights of another. The U.S. Constitution protects expression of your religious beliefs. If your interpretation includes abhorrence to abortion, then I see the Constitution protecting said belief, which protection logically would protect you from being forced to reap any benefit from the practice of abortion, no matter what a mortal priest might say about it. After all, in the world today are "priests" calling for the murder of "infidels" in the name of religion. Are we to look for mortals for interpretation of the Laws of God or do we look within?

My body is a "temple of God" for as long as I dwell within this temple God has given me. For me, to deliberately inject foul chemicals and known toxins, such as, but not limited to, aluminum and mercury, and formaldehyde, constitutes defiling my temple of God. To compel me to do so would, in my view, be an abhorrent violation of my expression of obedience to God.

This book makes a compelling case for the modern "Christian" to consider the controversy over forced vaccines from a personal religious perspective.

ENDORSEMENTS

The Divine Physician is Jesus Christ. All that is good flows from the Lord. I myself am not a medical professional, nor do I have any medical training or experience. I am, however, a father. As a father, the well-being of my own children is ever present in my mind: their education, their wellness, and their health.

In her book *Becoming Whole: Building Natural Immunity in the Body and Soul,* Lea Povozhaev presents a timely and important message about wellness. She adds her voice to the growing number of those concerned with the troubling, damaging misinformation propagated by our culture, which often informs the decisions parents make regarding the health of their families, including vaccination. There is a many-faceted discussion on vaccination. Added to this reality, is the current mood toward those who question vaccination. This mood is reflected in assumptions: "They are outsiders. They are not like us. They put the health of their children at extreme risk." In short, people who even question vaccination are often ostracized in our culture. What is worse, they are often degraded by some friends, extended family and medical professionals (and astonishingly even when they themselves are medical professionals!).

One of the most important foci in debates about vaccination should be the eradication of ideological methods of coercion. Truth must prevail and not the "versus" structure which divides. Dissemination of information can only be truly received without fear. Sometimes implementing actions derived from truthful information can be messy, just like life is often messy. Mrs. Povozhaev seeks with her work to offer a bright spot in the debate. To this end, she eloquently writes, "Becoming whole is preserving the sanctity of life by living whole and holy."

She offers for consideration many points for readers to discern in their own lives. She presents a plethora of information and stories from the lives of real people who have struggled through the issue of vaccination, and other health concerns, themselves. Through her own eyes and life, she offers the reader a piece of her own questions, struggles, and triumphs. She adds the perspective of this father, husband, and Orthodox priest to the testimonies of those who are navigating the precarious minefield of difficult choices in the American medical landscape. The greatest strength of her work is its character, which could be summed up in one word: Reflective.

Fr. Alexis Baldwin
Father, Husband, Priest in Charge at Holy Resurrection Orthodox Mission, North Augusta, SC

In the world today, our physical health is often thought of as an island, distanced from Creation, and what God meant for His beloved children. In *Becoming Whole: Building Natural Immunity in the Body and Soul* Lea Povozhaev shines light on areas of health that can blur the lines between secular and divine, and the holistic effect on our souls. I recommend reading *Becoming Whole: Building Natural Immunity in the Body and Soul* and to start reclaiming your health, and the health of your family, today.

Cynthia Damaskos
Author, *The Holistic Christian Woman*

Modern medicine has become a religion. It is not based on science. Dr. Robert Mendelsohn said it well: "Despite the tendency of doctors to call modern medicine an 'inexact science,' it is more accurate to say there is practically no science in modern medicine at all. Almost everything doctors do is based on a conjecture, a guess, a clinical impression, a whim, a hope, a wish, an opinion or a belief. In short, everything they do is based on anything but solid scientific evidence. Thus, medicine is not a science at all, but a belief system. Beliefs are held by every religion, including the Religion of Modern Medicine." Robert Mendelsohn, MD, Preface by Hans Ruesch, to 1000 Doctors (and many more) Against Vivisection.

"Thou shalt have no other gods before me" includes the "god" of modern medicine.
It is time that the belief system in vaccinations be challenged. Lea Povozhaev has done this in her book *Becoming Whole: Building Natural Immunity in the Body and Soul*. I highly recommend reading it.

Barbara F. Gregory
Independent researcher http://barbfeick.com/vaccinations
A Study of the Association of Vaccinations and Injections with Food Allergies

DEDICATION

The following is dedicated to Viktor, Dominik, Elizabeth, Galina, Alexis, and children everywhere:

O God, our heavenly father, Who lovest mankind and art most merciful and compassionate, have mercy upon thy servants, Viktor, Dominik, Elizabeth, and Galina[1], for whom I humbly pray to thee, and commend to thy gracious care and protection. Be thou, O God, their guide and guardian in all their endeavors, lead them in the path of thy truth, and draw them nearer to thee that they may lead a godly and righteous life in thy love and fear, doing thy will in all things. Give them grace that they may be temperate, industrious, diligent, devout and charitable. Defend them against the assaults of the enemy, and grant them wisdom and strength to resist all temptation and corruption of this life, and direct them in the way of salvation, through the merits of thy Son, our Savior Jesus Christ, and the intercessions of His Holy Mother and thy blessed Saints. Amen.

****

'Body' and 'soul' are the constituents of human existence; the Orthodox emphasis on the Resurrection confirms its view that human life and human fulfillment are inextricably bound to both the physical and the spiritual dimensions of human existence. In more contemporary terms, body and personhood are essential for the fulfillment of human potential.[2]

---

1   The following is a prayer for children and one may replace the names here with the children for whom one prays.
2   Antoniades, 1:204-208 qtd. in Fr. Stanley Harakas, "For the Health of Body and Soul: An Eastern Orthodox Introduction to Bioethics," http://www.goarch.org/ourfaith/ourfaith8076, *Greek Orthodox Archdiocese of America*, 2015, web, 01 July 2015.

INTRODUCTION

I am an Orthodox Christian mother of five children. My first two children are vaccinated, three are not. My children without their shots are healthier with fewer colds, flu, ear infections, etc. When a sickness befalls them, it usually clears quickly. I do not support vaccination, and I do support holistic health—living whole and holy. Living holistically is a pro-life journey. The Orthodox Church is pro-life. I love the Church. Her Truth, Love, and Life saves us. The second edition of this book is endorsed by the Church with the intention to share the Truth with its followers. This book offers readers information to questions concerning fetal stem cells and vaccines, and it looks at this complicated issue in light of the whole person: body and soul. This work is timely, as the Holy Synod will soon convene to discuss vaccination. I have engaged this work prayerfully. Theotokos, save us!

In *Becoming Whole: Building Natural Immunity in the Body and Soul,* the message is on preserving the sanctity of life by deliberate care for the body and spirit. The first half of the book is concerned with holistic health care, calling for a need to consider individuals' unique bodies and souls and work with nature by building the immune system through nutrition and healthy lifestyles, and especially on the necessity of reconsidering the dangerous practice of vaccination. My argument's premise is on the sanctity of life: not using vaccines cultured with aborted fetal stem cells (as over 23 current vaccines are), and not vaccinating because toxic preservatives and harmful adjuvants poison the body.

1. Since the late 1800s, animals have been used in the production of vaccines, but this is less desirable to human cells from aborted babies. The availability and care of live animals is less convenient than the use of cells from aborted babies; additionally, animals carry other bacteria and viruses and have contaminated vaccines (i.e. polio in 1960s). Some viruses don't grow well in animal cells. The use of aborted fetuses for vaccine development is touted a great medical advancement.

2. From the 1960s to present, research and development of vaccines uses hundreds of aborted babies (i.e. Planned Parenthood recently sold organs to pharmaceutical companies, whose biggest market is vaccines.) After a time, most human cells cease replication and new abortions are considered necessary. Trace amounts of fetal cells are in vaccines when cultured in such cells.

3. Vaccination is not the lesser of two evils because vaccines are not protective; the immunological response measured is the presence of antibodies, which a body produces to the foreign invasion of a virus, but this doesn't make one safe from illness—it causes harm in the body by compromising the immune system with unnaturally injecting toxins and viruses.

USA & CANADA - ABORTED FETAL CELL LINE PRODUCTS AND ETHICAL ALTERNATIVES
(Nov 2017) References

Disease	Product Name	Manufacturer	Fetal Cell Line	Ethical Version	Manufacturer	Cell Line
Acute Respiratory	Adenovirus 4,7 Oral	Barr Labs	WI-38	None	N/A	N/A
Chickenpox	All Varivax, Varilrix	Merck, GSK	WI-38, MRC-5	None	N/A	N/A
Cystic Fibrosis	Pulmozyme	Genentech	HEK-293	N-acetylcysteine, Hypersal	Various	N/A
Anemia (Cancer patients, severe kidney disease)	Procrit, Epoetin alfa Epogen, Aranesp, Darbepoetin alfa	Amgen	Human erythropoietin gene from fetal liver lambda.hE1/	None	N/A	N/A
Ebola - In Development	NIAID/GSK ChAd3 AdVacEbola VSV-EBOV	GSK J&J/Crucell, NewLink /BioProtSv	Procell92/HEK-293 PER C6, HEK-293	rVSV-ZEBOV-GP GOVOX-E301, E-302 ZMapp Therapeutic	Merck/New Link GeoVax LeafBio	Vero Chick eggs Tobacco
Heart problems	Abciximab (Repro)	Eli Lilly	HEK-293	Integrilin, Angiomax	Merck, Medicine Co.	N/A
Hemophilia	rhFVI, VIII, Eloctate	Octapharma, BioGen	HEK-293	Advate, Kogenate	Baxter	Hamster
Hepatitis A	Vaqta, Havrix Avaxim, Epaxal	Merck, GSK Sanofi, Berna	MRC-5 MRC-5	Aimmugen None in US or Canada	Kaketsuken (Japan, Asia & Europe)	Vero (monkey)
Hepatitis A & B Hepatitis A & Typhoid	Twinrix Vivaxim	GSK Sanofi	MRC-5 MRC-5	Engerix Hep-B Only Recombivax Hep-B, TyphimVi	GSK Merck	Yeast Yeast
Infection prevention	G-CSF	Octapharma	HEK-293	Neupogen, Zarxio	Amgen, Sandoz	E-coli
Measles/Mumps/ Rubella	MMR, Priorix	Merck, GSK	RA273, WI-38, MRC-5	MR+M (Japan only)	Kitasato Daiichi Sankyo	Hen, rabbit
Measles-Rubella	MR Vax, Eolarix	Merck, GSK.	RA273, WI-38, MRC-5	Attenuvax (Measles Only)* MR (Japan only)	Merck Kitasato Daiichi Sankyo	Hen eggs Hen, rabbit
Mumps-Rubella	Biavax II	Merck	RA273, WI-38	Mumpsvax (Mumps	Merck	Hen eggs
Rubella	Meruvax II	Merck	RA273, WI-38	Takahashi (Japan only)	Kitasato Daiichi Sankyo	Rabbit
MMR + Chickenpox	ProQuad/MMR-V Priorix Tetra	Merck GSK	RA273, WI-38, MRC-5	None	N/A	N/A
Polio	Poliovax, DT PolAds Polio Sabin (oral)	Sanofi Pasteur GSK	MRC-5 MRC-5	IPOL, IMOVAX® Polio**	Sanofi Pasteur	Vero
Polio Combination (DTaP + polio+ HiB)	Pentacel, Quadracel Infanrix-IPV-HiB	Sanofi Pasteur GSK	MRC-5	Pediacel, Pediarix, Any HiB DTap, IPOL, Infanrix Hexa, Kinrix	Sanofi, GSK	Vero
Rabies	Imovax**	Sanofi Pasteur	MRC-5	RabAvert	Novartis	Hen eggs
Rheumatoid Arthritis	Enbrel	Amgen	WI-26 VA4 - RDNA	Humira, Cimzia, Orencia	Abbott, UCB, BMS	Hamster
Shingles	Zostavax	Merck.	WI-38, MRC-5	Shingrix	GSK	Hamster
Smallpox	Acambis 1000	Acambis	MRC-5	ACAM2000, MVA3000	Acambis/Baxter	Vero

Chart Reference Information:

Note: Immune-Globulin shots will provide temporary immunity (4-6 months) for Hepatitis-A and Rubella (3-4 months)

*Moral versions of Measles and Mumps are currently UNAVAILABLE as of January 2010 – TELL MERCK TO PROVIDE THEM!

**NOTE: IMOVAX®Polio is a moral version for polio vaccine in Canada and is not the same as IMOVAX for rabies.

ANY VACCINE NOT LISTED ABOVE DOES NOT USE ABORTED FETAL CELL LINES

Copy Permissible with Credit Children of God for Life ©

Here are the bare bones, though this "beast" mutates and grows larger. There are 73 vaccines in the recommended schedule. The CDC provides detailed charts with this public information. Keep in mind that many vaccines are combined into one injection. Of these recommended childhood vaccines, at least 23 are cultured using fetal stem cells. Additionally, hundreds of babies have been aborted in vaccine development.

The chart[3] here is from Children of God for Life, founded by Dr. Theresa Deisher, world renowned stem cell scientist and Catholic Christian. This list is a comprisal of vaccines using fetal stem cells. While it is suggested here that there are "ethical alternatives," I argue that there can be no such possibility. Vaccines that do not use fetal stem cells in their production still use cells of other animals such as hens, chickens, monkeys, hamsters, rabbits, etc. There are also harmful preservatives and antigens in the formulation for the vaccine to be used. Tobacco, yeast, and E-coli are in vaccines. No ethical alternative exists when such ingredients harm the body. Immune systems are compromised when vaccines are injected into a human's deep muscle tissue where vaccine material does enter the bloodstream in trace amounts. To be clear, vaccines cross the brain-blood barrier. Their toxicity has a cumulative effect. By age five, 51 doses are to be given to a child. That is 51 times the amount of heavy metals, DNA fragments, formaldehyde, etc. While people are told that these toxicities are minute, many people have negative reactions, some initially, others after a time, even years.

Medical research published in PMC in various scientific articles states: "Three cell substrates, human diploid cells, continuous cell lines and primary cell lines, are always used for developing vaccines."[4]

Bo Ma, et al. state that there were 80 elective abortions involved in the research and final production of the current rubella vaccine: 21 abortions from the original WI-1 through WI-26 fetal cell lines that failed, plus WI-38 itself, plus 67 from the attempts to isolate the rubella virus. Some who believe in the usefulness of vaccines but do not support abortion would desire vaccines using adult stem cells or stem cells from placentas and umbilical cords; however, embryonic fetal stem cells are pluripotent, which means that they can become all cell types in the body. This is most useful for the research and cultivation of vaccines.

In a PubMed article on diploid cells (WI-38, MRC-5) titled: "Vaccines, biotechnology and their connection with induced abortion," the abstract states that "[v]accines have their origin in induced abortions. Among these vaccines we find the following: rubella, measles, mumps, rabies, polio, smallpox, hepatitis A, chickenpox, and herpes zoster.

---

[3] "USA and Canada – Aborted Fetal Cell Line Products and Ethical Alternatives (Nov. 2017)," https://cogforlife.org/wp-content/uploads/vaccineListOrigFormat.pdf .
[4] Ma, Bo, et al, "Characteristics and viral propagation properties of a new human diploid cell line, walvax-2, and its suitability as a candidate cell substrate for vaccine production," https://www.ncbi.nlm.nih.gov/pmc/articles/PMC4526920, Human Vaccines and Immunotherapeutics, 24 Mar. 2015, web 31 Jan. 2018.

Nowadays, other abortion tainted vaccines cultivated on transformed cells (293, PER.C6) are in the pipeline: flu, Respiratory Syncytial and parainfluenza viruses, HIV, West Nile virus, Ebola, Marburg and Lassa, hepatitis B and C, foot and mouth disease, Japanese encephalitis, dengue, tuberculosis, anthrax, plague, tetanus and malaria." While not all these vaccines are in the childhood recommended schedule, people are encouraged to get vaccinated throughout life.[5]

Many of us are unaware that vaccines were introduced after diseases were on the decline and have never lessened illness, ever. In fact, since the beginning of vaccination in the 1900s, doctors, scientists, parents, and care-takers have warned that vaccines render us susceptible to food allergies and eczema, diseases they are supposed to prevent, and compromise one's overall-health in numerous ways including cancer and infertility. Vaccination is especially dangerous in vulnerable populations such as children and the ill with immature and or weak immune systems, and even those who are healthy and vaccinated shed viruses after vaccination. Society is healthier when vaccine free. Healthy societies have clean water and food and systems of sanitation so that people are not living in filth. And yet, oftentimes, we offer third-world countries vaccines (which we buy from China with horribly lax safety checks) and do not offer them the true key to wellness. Throughout history—from the smallpox vaccine in the 1800s to the polio vaccines in the 1950s, to all other vaccines—vaccination has contributed to increase in diseases, infections, and viruses, as well as neurologic and immune disorders. There is an astronomical increase in vaccines, and this profits pharmaceutical companies. Government and institutions of higher learning are often granted large sums of funding from pharmaceutical companies to ensure that law and research is in their favor. In the 1980s, 20 vaccines were recommended for children, and today, 2016, there are 73 recommended vaccinations by the time one is 18. By 2025, there are plans for 300 vaccines, and, if we allow it, these will be mandated. Some argue this is a return to the Dark Ages.

Becoming Whole: Building Natural Immunity in the Body and Soul, is a book with a message of hope. Good ultimately triumphs, and life continues on. In the second portion of the book, I reflect on faith in God and experiences in the body. Prayer is my focus here, and it is living, interactive, life-giving and life-sustaining. Prayer reflects one's relationship with God, and by prayer a person more deeply realizes herself and the meaning of life. Today, practices such as secular meditation differ from prayer, and I discuss and illustrate with real-life stories how seeking God and seeking self-go together powerfully, revealing more of our character than any meditation outside of God could enable. At the end, illness and death as one's saving road reflects upon the fact that wellness and illness can both develop personhood, but only through the common touchstone of the sanctity of life.

---

[5] Calderon, Redondo, https://www.ncbi.nlm.nih.gov/m/pubmed/18611078/?i=6&from=WI-38+vaccine, May-Aug. 2008, web 31 Jan. 2018.

I have an urgent, specific message on vaccines and worship of self instead of true prayer—as both are falsehoods in the name of wellness. To be whole and holy begins from within the body, and always in relationship with God. In *Becoming Whole: Building Natural Immunity in the Body and Soul*, reflections on experiences in my body in relationship to my faith in God are intended to show why I questioned medical science. To these ends, the first half of this book is on vaccination and health care, and the second half reflects on my personal journey of faith—a process unique to my life: my body, mind, and soul, but in common with all others also seeking to realize faith. This book is a reminder that realizing faith occurs through our bodies. Accordingly, prayer is understood in *Becoming Whole: Building Natural Immunity in the Body and Soul* beyond recitation or Bible reading. Prayer is living, and it occurs through one's very body and soul.

Seeking the Truth is tied to my personal relationship with God. I wish to persuade others to question the practice of vaccination in relationship to faith in the Giver of Life and Source of Truth. My argument's premise is on the sanctity of life: not using vaccines with aborted fetal stem cells, and not vaccinating because toxins and harmful adjuvants poison the body. Learning to become more well is a process, and today's social norms must be re-examined. I do so from an Orthodox Christian perspective, and so the second half of my current book reflects on my personal faith journey in chapters that address topics such as meditation, prayer, and death.

This is not just another anti-vaccination book.

It is a Christian's spiritual journey towards Truth, which, I believe, is realized in the body. Just as one is taught about God and then has the accountability to follow Him, the first half of my book teaches of the many ills of vaccination with the expectation that readers will consider the second portion on other topics (in relationship to the first part) and deepen their appreciation for tending personhood: body and spirit.

This is not just another account of one's spiritual journey.

Orthodox Christianity is deeply satisfying, challenging, and fulfilling. I see no reason to re-invent the wheel in my desire for body-spirit unity, as the ancient faith has always been about whole personhood, becoming holy as God is. Spirituality today often misplaces God and one's physical and spiritual relationship to Him. Obedience to God is life giving and edifies the soul of human beings. I share my faith to explore living, breathing love of God, and to communicate the authentic struggles of living faithfully in today's society, particularly where practices such as vaccination threaten the sanctity of life. This is more than an argument for Orthodoxy. *Becoming Whole: Building Natural Immunity in the Body and Soul* is a call to honor life and seek Truth. If we do, it is up to God to help each along one's unique journey. In the body, I seek my soul.

Other arguments have been made concerning one's civil liberties, the history and future of vaccination, and scientific explanations of various vaccines and their effects on individuals. While I address this research as part of my reasoning against vaccines, the fresh and essential message that I have is that God is Life and that which is good fosters life. True wellness is becoming more whole and holy. My book is a journey towards Truth regarding wellness.

My ten-year-old asked, "Why does it matter what others choose to do with their bodies? People can do what they choose." I mentioned to my thoughtful, growing boy that what others' choose to do with their bodies and the bodies of their children matters for all of us.

"What happens if you were to marry someone and she has cancer in her thirties? Or, what if you and she cannot have children? Would you want to pay taxes for costly health care that many will require because of chronic diseases, syndromes, and autoimmune disorders? Would it trouble you to observe a society where more than half are in some way neurologically impaired?" He understood. I hope that readers likewise consider the high cost of our current vaccination program. May society embark upon a journey towards holistic wellness that includes living more whole and holy in honor of the Giver of Life.

I wish to alert Christians, among others who value the sanctity of life, of one of the serious failings of the health care industry. People are confused and even beguiled by health care and drug industries that promote an endless array of commercials for every conceivable medication during the national news every night. Drugs are advertised for aging baby-boomers who are dealing with everything from arthritis to hormonal imbalances and seeking remedies through prescription. Many other drugs are touted to alleviate symptoms of depression, mental distraction, and sexual enhancement, and parents are conditioned to believe that their family's answers rest in the hands of "Mother-Pharma." There is a serious lack of understanding for life cycles that cannot, and should not, be exchanged for prescription "cure-alls." The potential side effects of such drugs may be worse than the symptoms the meds are attempting to alleviate.

Christians expect problems, complications, and deceptions in a fallen world. It is difficult to know how to attain wellness, which is wholeness and holiness, in our lives. Western health care promotes medication as a powerful tool for wellness. It is a lie, evidenced by our own lives and those around us who do not seem healthy, happy, or well. While Christians accept this condition in a fallen world, perhaps we should not accept suffering that is a direct result of pharmaceutical companies profiting at the expense of human beings' lives. When it is possible, taking a more natural and holistic approach to health will help us in countless ways. A good place to begin is a mind-change from thinking that medication = health, to understanding how proper nutrition and positive lifestyles = health. This would lessen many needless drugs, surgeries, health, and financial complications.

A paradigm shift is needed. Shots and pills can't make us well. Food and lifestyle is key to the state of one's health. Medications are abundant, and despite likely side effects, many are taking them with a false confidence in their ability to make us well. I have been ridiculed for not taking painkillers after giving birth, "don't try to be a martyr," a nurse said, but she failed to understand that my body was not in pain that necessitated the drug, and taking it would likely constipate me. In our culture of taking Tylenol for aches and pains, it takes an open mind to try another way. For example, sometimes a fever is better treated with a cool rag on the forehead and by allowing the body to have a rise in temperature and naturally heal itself. Miraculously, the body is able to heal itself, and it will become stronger in doing so naturally. Many livers have been damaged by the "gentle" drug Tylenol, even prescribed for infants after vaccines, which certainly should not be administered to babies after their shots because of their body's enormous job working out the injected toxins from the vaccines. Understanding why it benefits us to heal with fewer pharmaceuticals is at the center of the switch to caring for our health holistically.

As a culture, we believe in medication to take away pain, to cure illness, and to prevent disease. With our faith in medicine, there tends to be denial of the very real consequences of taking drugs into our bodies. There continues a surge in medications, including vaccines. In the U.S., there is a ridiculous increase in vaccines and doses of various vaccines (in the form of booster shoots given after a period of time when the original vaccine is no longer effecting "immunity")—from 16 vaccines and 70 doses 3 years ago. Now, this number steadily increases, with recommendations from the CDC added to the childhood list of vaccines as states prepare bills for mandatory vaccination. Recently, added to the 70, are two vaccines for meningitis, and the HPV vaccine is now recommended for nine year olds, though this is a vaccine for cervical cancer caused by sexual activity.

I see health problems in youth, and fear another ten years will increase these growing problems. For example, I teach Composition at a local community college, and a student presented on autism. She is autistic, as is her boyfriend, and in a class of 25, seven additional students rose their hands when I asked if they have someone close to them who suffers with autism. A mother, whose son was diagnosed at three with autism, says she and her husband wonder if there are just more diagnoses. The term "autism" has been in use since 1908 with a history of development, but there is no denying that there are many more children on the autism spectrum today than any other time in history.

Dr. Andrew Wakefield, whose reputation was intentionally smeared and whose research was and is denied by powerful groups, argued vaccines as being a cause of autism twenty years ago.[6] His news was thrown out, and vaccines continued for most.

6   Dr. Joseph Mercola, "Dr. Andrew Wakefield's Interview on His MMR Study: Why Medical Authorities Went to Such Extremes to Silence Dr. Andrew Wakefield,"

Health problems, including autism, persist. The fact is, the vaccine industry is a huge market, and its astronomical profits are for the pharmaceutical companies and the U.S. government.[7] "For example, did you know that the U.S. Department of Health and Human Services has accumulated $3.5 BILLION in vaccine tax revenue which is currently 'sitting' in the Vaccine Injury Compensation Trust Fund?" Since 1986, Congress granted legal immunity to drug companies. They could not be sued by anyone harmed by vaccines. They did not need to make their vaccines safer or more effective. In 1988, a $0.75 excise tax was put on vaccines the CDC recommends. The taxpayer funds compensation for vaccine-related injury or death that can be "proven" as caused by the vaccine(s). Many are in court for over ten years and very few are granted compensation. The Vaccine Injury Compensation Trust Fund has grown large because 'autism' has been taken off the list of vaccine injuries that can be compensated for from this fund. By March 1, 2010, 13,330 cases had been filed in the special vaccine court, with 5,617 representing autism cases. Of those 13,330 cases filed up to March 1, 2010, only 2,409 were compensated. [....] Dr. William Thompson of the CDC has become a whistleblower and admitted that one of the main studies used to supposedly 'prove' there is no link between the MMR [measles/mumps/rubella] vaccine and autism did not follow study protocol, and withheld contradicting data showing an increase in autism among some groups, particularly African American boys.

Despite the obvious correlation between increased vaccines and autism, if autism were seen as vaccine-related harm, the government would lose a ton of money. Currently, many people are revisiting Dr. Wakefield's claims.

People deserve the right to make informed decisions concerning their bodies and the bodies of their parents, children, and other loved ones. I believe that this is much more than a political issue, just as abortion, euthanasia, and homosexuality are more than mere politics to Christians. The body and the spirit are two undivided components of personhood. In the fourth century, Emperor Constantine unearthed Christ's Cross during the Christian Revolution in Byzantium. Miracles of healing occurred by Christ's cross. The people's national anthem was a prayer: "O Lord, save Thy people and bless Thine inheritance. Grant victory to the Orthodox kings over the barbarians!" Faith was realized in the very lives of a nation's people, and the result was Elevation of the Life-giving Cross, a Christian feast still revered by Orthodox Christians in September. Politics and faith are in ways bound up together, and laws that govern a land evidence the state of a people's collective conscience. Christians are being pushed back into the catacombs of current America, and there is direct attack on the sanctity of life.

http://articles.mercola.com/sites/articles/archive/2010/04/10/wakefield-interview.aspx, Mercola, 10 April 2010, web, 01 Sept. 2015.

7 The following information comes from: "How the Government has Earned 3.5 BILLION from the Claim that Vaccines Don't Cause Autism," http://healthimpactnews.com/2014/how-the-government-has-earned-3-5-billion-from-the-claim-that-vaccines-dont-cause-autism/, Health Impact News, 17 Sept. 2014. Web, 01 Sept. 2015.

A New York Russian Orthodox mom won the right to exempt her autistic son from getting the school-mandated MMR vaccination after citing her moral opposition to abortion.[8] The woman said she objected on religious grounds because the MMR vaccine includes fetal stem cells from aborted fetuses.[9] During the summer and fall of 2013, the city Department of Education rejected her bid for exemption after questioning the sincerity of her religious beliefs, but the mother filed an appeal. After the mother "produced information relative to specific ingredients" that showed the vaccine included aborted fetal stem cells, an education commissioner granted the child exemption. The law currently provides for a religious exemption that is documented in writing and "heartfelt." The mother argued that;

[A]bortion is clearly considered a mortal sin and is [an] abhorrent act to any Christian. [....] The vaccine manufacturers' use of aborted fetal cells in its products and research means that I cannot associate with them or support them financially (by buying their products), for such support would make me complicit to their sin and answerable to God for this violation.

City health officials denied the mother's request because they said the Russian Orthodox Church had not taken a strong stand against student vaccinations.

Once the truth begins to unravel, the picture is impossible to deny. Vaccines, as they are currently administered, are for profit not health, and they violate the sanctity of life. With the plan to mandate vaccination, we are at risk both physically and spiritually, if we consider certain important facts. Spiritually, if I am aware that a vaccine includes aborted fetal stem cells using this vaccine, it is a sin against Life. An Orthodox Christian understanding of salvation is that it is a process of becoming like God in every way other than "essence."[10] Personhood is both body and spirit to an Orthodox Christian. Though we will become ill and die, as good stewards, we preserve the life, which God allows us. Mandating vaccination concerns me as a Christian for many reasons, spiritual and physical, as stated above, and many more, as I will explain in this book. I hope that as the Church becomes more aware of the current vaccination program in the United States, the faithful and our spiritual leaders will take a strong stand against the current practice of vaccination.

For this to happen, the faithful will need to learn about the current practice of vaccination in the U.S., including ingredients of vaccines, rates of childhood diseases and

8   "NY Mom Wins Right to not Vaccinate Son over Religious Belief," http://nypost.com/2015/08/31/anti-abortion-mom-wins-right-to-not-vaccinate-her-autistic-son/, *New York Post*, 31 August 2015, web, 31 August 2015.
9   For a list of vaccines using fetal stem cells, see "Aborted Fetal Cell Line Products and Ethical Alternatives (August 2015)," https://www.cogforlife.org/vaccineListOrigFormat.pdf, *Children of God for Life*, Aug. 2015, web, 01 Sept. 2015. In addition to the use of fetal stem cell line products, vaccines include harmful adjuvants and ingredients such as peanut oil that can lead to allergy and autoimmune diseases.
10   Fr. John Matusiak, personal correspondence, August 31, 2015.

disorders compared to other nations, and probe information that is available from sources that the pharmaceutical companies do not fund (which takes us to information not sponsored / censored by the U.S. government and institutions of higher learning, in many cases). Unfortunately, we have not been told by our doctors that most current vaccines are cultured in aborted fetal stem cells (and include trace amounts of fetal stem cells); the ingredients are not readily shared with parents. Many more vaccines are being developed using aborted fetuses,[11] and I wonder where the Christian outrage is concerning this reality. This matters for Christians because we value life. Aborted fetuses have no place in our bodies. In fact, many vaccines today contain unavoidable traces of fetal cells, and the injection of foreign DNA into human bodies is arguably causing many adverse effects, including autism.[12] It is ironic that vaccines are an assault on the sanctity of life, considering we have been led to believe that vaccines protect us from disease and preserve our lives. The current program of vaccination in the U.S. is a network of deceit predicated on the premise of profit in the name of health.

The Orthodox Church is pro-life. Fr. John Matusiak shared the following sentiment in an e-mail correspondence with me where he discussed the Church's large presence at the March for Life in D.C. this year, Metropolitan Tikhon's message on the Sanctity of Life, as well as the Metropolitan's prayer before the March: "One can hardly conclude that the Church's leaders do anything other than support the pro-life message—and this has been the norm for decades."

The U.S. government and heath care is wrapped up together. There is a federal excise tax per each recommended childhood vaccine, and the information is plain as day—straight from the United States Centers for Disease Control and Prevention.[13] Former CDC director, Julie Gerberding, recently sold 38,368 shares of Merck Stock for $2.3 million.[14] Health care is a business negatively affecting the health of society. It is difficult to believe, but impossible to deny when researchers (much of which remains outside of the mainstream media, but of late voices of doctors, scholars, and whistleblowers argue against vaccines even within mainstream media) present clear and persuasive scientific facts that explain how vaccines are related to what we can clearly see in society, often in our own families, concerning an increase in viral infections, neurological problems, affective and autoimmune disorders, and allergies.

11 The government and our health care system is wrapped up together: Ertelt, Steven, "Obama Sends $1 Million to Planned Parenthood in Three States After It Sells Aborted Baby Parts," http://www.LifeNews.com/2015/09/02/obama-sends-1-million-to-planned-parenthood-in-three-states-after-it-sells-aborted-baby-parts/, Life News, 02 Sept. 2015, web, 05 Sept. 2015.
12 Matt, "Fetal Stem Cells and Foreign DNA in Vaccines," http://www.dinnerforthought.com/blog/why-dont-you-vaccinate, Dinner for Thought Blog, 17 Oct. 2015, web, 20 Oct. 2015.
13 "Vaccines for Children: Current CDC Vaccine Price List," http://www.cdc.gov/vaccines/programs/vfc/awardees/vaccine-management/price-list/, U.S. Department of Health and Human Services, 01 Oct. 2015, web, 02 Oct. 2015.
14 "Former CDC Director Julie Gerberding sells 38,368 shares of Merck Stock for $2.3 Million," http://healthimpactnews.com/2015/former-cdc-director-julie-gerberding-sells-38368-shares-of-merck-stock-for-2-3-million/, Health Impact News, 01 Oct. 2015, web, 01 Oct. 2015.

Fear of God is the beginning of wisdom. We must also fear to go against Life. We are created to love the Lord, the Giver of Life. I hope, pray, and appeal to all Christians to stand against the current program of vaccination because of its use of aborted fetuses. This would provide a stronger case for religious exemptions to vaccination. At the least, it is important to protect the right of exemption for those who think that the risks of vaccination out-weigh the benefits, whether the risks are understood as harm to the body and or harm to the soul.

The message of *Becoming Whole: Building Natural Immunity in the Body and Soul* is a call to Christians to preserve the sanctity of life by deliberate care for the body and soul. While recipes and how-to books are helpful, this book does not define the way to be well. Instead, in light of my own experiences, observations, and research, I argue that life in Christ is a process of realizing that the body and spirit are integrated and what we do in the body matters for our souls. My perspective is as an Orthodox Christian who is struggling to navigate faith in the world. The issue of vaccination is my central illustration of the disconnect between the body and soul that we currently engage. I also discuss life as a prayer and prayer versus secular meditation practices gaining popularity in our times because these topics are likewise about seeking wellness through reintegration of the body and soul, necessary in order that we may become more whole. Though the Church has not taken a stance on vaccination, this is because many faithful do not know that fetal stem cells are used in the production of vaccines (among other disturbing facts). The Orthodox Church states that in no case is the use of fetal stem cells acceptable for Orthodox Christians. Back in 2001, the Holy Synod of the Orthodox Church in America issued a statement that in no case is the use of fetal stem cells acceptable for Orthodox Christians. Furthermore, as defenders of the Giver of Life, the Church has a responsibility to continue its deliberations over the very meaning and value of human life.

We cannot, however, condone the manipulation of embryonic cells in any form for research purposes, including lines developed from destroyed embryos. Rather, we can only express dismay at the fact that the debate over this issue has avoided major considerations regarding the very meaning and value of human life.[15]

It is time for unnecessary suffering to stop. The issue of vaccination is integral to faith in the Giver of Life, the Lord, and the only reason Christians have for silence is ignorance to the ingredients and the results of injecting harmful adjuvants and fetal stem cells into tiny bodies. It is time to give voice to the babies who will be aborted with the intent of using their lives in medical research for the "greater good," which is a lie in and of itself. Vaccination harms. Period. Research into the history and current practice reveals this

---

[15] "Embryonic Stem Cell Research in the Perspective of Orthodox Christianity," OCA Chancery, https://oca.org/holy-synod/statements/holy-synod/embryonic-stem-cell-research-in-the-perspective-of-orthodox-christianity, The Orthodox Church in America Chancery, Syosset, N.Y., 17 Oct. 2001, web, 6 Feb. 2018.

truth, and if one is willing to honestly weigh the evidence presented, my research will demonstrate why we must reconsider vaccination.

The Holy Spirit, the Lord, the Giver of Life, reveals Himself through unexpected life situations, even tragedy. Nevertheless, it is better when suffering can be stopped because one is willing to open the mind and reconsider vaccination. It isn't difficult to notice that there is a disconnect between expectations for health and realities following current practices in health care, particularly concerning vaccines and over-medication. Nine years earlier, Orthodox Christian priest, Fr. Alexis Baldwin[16], logically predicted that people would endorse the use of fetal stem cells from aborted babies in vaccines to "save lives." At this earlier point in time, the use of fetal stem cells in vaccination was said to be an isolated incident. Fr. Baldwin argues that there is now a corporate mechanism in place: the abortion and medical industries together with pharmaceutical companies encourage women to abort and donate the fetuses to medical research. Today, movements such as "I heart my abortion" and "Shout your abortion," are marks of a time where death is celebrated. Within this anti-Christ culture, the ethics of vaccination do not concern many. Worse yet, there is no way to formulate vaccines with safe and effective ingredients that would not include animal stem cells and dangerous adjuvants. This is so because the ingredients in the vaccines are necessary to produce the antigen effect of the vaccine in one's body. "If Christians remain silent, who will speak out?" asks Fr. Baldwin. He adds that we trust companies to put good ingredients in medicines and are scandalized that life has been taken and fetuses destroyed for medical research.

We are being fed an enormous lie that has oppressed the truth since the beginning.[17] There most certainly are fetal stem cells and trace amounts of foreign human DNA[18] in vaccines, and even the ingredients listed on the vaccine inserts include this information. Whether one is uncomfortable with that reality—that baby cells are injected into babies—my argument is this: What profits the body, profits the soul. While the soul is growing and can profit even in illness and death, God wills that every human being preserve the sanctity of life to the degree that one is aware and able.

What is good for the body also profits the soul because wholeness and holiness are synergistic. I began my quest into vaccination with interest in the benefit / harm to the body. I have found that building the body and feeding the spirit occurs by building natural immunity and not by vaccination. Not surprisingly, the soul also benefits from building natural immunity because vaccines from their inception have been steeped in

16 Baldwin, Fr. Alexis, parish priest, Holy Resurrection Orthodox Mission, North Augusta, personal correspondence, 03 Oct. 2015.
17 "What You Didn't Know About the Aborted Baby Parts in Your Vaccines—Living Whole," http://www.livingwhole.org/what-you-didnt-know-about-the-aborted-baby-parts-in-your-vaccines/, Living Whole, 14 Sept. 2015, web, 07 Oct. 2015.
18 "Autism and Cancer Related to Human Fetal DNA in Vaccines. Study," Global Research News, 19 Sept. 2014, web, 07 Oct. 2015.

deception. Vaccines have been said to save lives and keep well, but this is not true. In fact, women have been cajoled into abortions for the rubella vaccine, among others. Currently, there are vaccines in production using fetal stem cells, and Planned Parenthood is selling baby parts as in-tact as possible to pharmaceutical companies. Sadly, MRC-5 and WI-38 fetal stem cell lines, used in the production of vaccines, were healthy second trimester pregnancies that were aborted for "social reasons."[19] The abortions for those fetal cell lines were done with the intent to make vaccines. This is explained on *Children of God for Life*, under the tab for "vaccines and abortion." Many mistakenly have heard that there were two aborted babies used in the production of vaccines, and this occurred in the 1960s. Sadly, hundreds of aborted babies are used in one vaccine production. While fetal cells replicate more than other cells, new "material" is required for medical research and drug production, which abortions provide.[20]

Many have researched vaccines, and my work shares vital information of which too few of us are aware. Details such as the ingredients of our vaccines[21], the fact that cells used in the production of vaccines come from human tumors (called "human diploid cells")[22,23], and since the 1970s autoimmune disorders and injection-site tumors have been associated with the use of vaccines.[24] I ask for others to consider the following information and with courage to believe the Truth. We must unite in our prayers to God to protect our children. I ask that others read the research and consider carefully the cautionary tales that informed individuals provide for no reason other than their commitment to the holistic wellness of human beings. Consider the hard truth in light of society, despite having been told lies that have grown comfortable. May we change our minds with faith in God for the salvation of our souls, and for the effect, our actions may then have in this world.

By one's choice for God, one wills for life instead of death. Death exists because mankind turned away from God. Death is not punishment from God. Death of the soul is

---

19 *Children of God for Life: The Pro-Life World Leader in the Campaign for Ethical Vaccines, Medications and Consumer Products*, https://cogforlife.org/vaccines-abortions/, Children of God, 2015, web, 01 Oct. 2015.

20 Azvolinsky, Anna, "Of Cells and Limits," http://www.the-scientist.com/?articles.view%2FarticleNo%2F42256%2Ftitle%2FOf-Cells-and-Limits%2F, The Scientist Magazine, 01 Mar. 2015, web, 07 Oct. 2015.

21 *Children of God for Life: The Pro-Life World Leader in the Campaign for Ethical Vaccines, Medications and Consumer Products*, https://www.cogforlife.org/vaccineListOrigFormat.pdf, Children of God, 2015, web, 01 Oct. 2015.

22 "Blood, Vaccines and Other Biologics," http://www.fda.gov/downloads/AdvisoryCommittees/CommitteesMeetingMaterials/BloodVaccinesandOther Biologics/VaccinesandRelatedBiologicalProductsAdvisoryCommittee/UCM319573.pdf, Federal Drug Administration, 15 April 2015, web, 07 Oct. 2015.

23 B, Ma, et. al., "Characteristics and viral propagation properties of a new human diploid cell line, Walvax-2, and its suitability as a candidate cell substrate for vaccine production," http://www.ncbi.nlm.nih.gov/m/pubmed/25803132/, PubMed, 2015, web, 07 Oct. 2015.

24 Fields, Bernard, MD, "Genetic Manipulation of Reovirus—A Model for Modification of Disease?," http://www.nejm.org/doi/full/10.1056/NEJM197211162872007, NEJM, 16 Nov. 1972, web, 07 Oct. 2015.

a result of sin that separates a person from the Giver and Sustainer of all Life. The wages of sin are death. All bodies die, but for those who will, Christ saves. Jesus Christ "tramples down death by death, and upon those in the tomb bestows life."[25] Vile death is conquered. Here and now, we pass through illness and death but take heart because He has overcome the world and all its sufferings. Life, and its intended fullness, is the reality to which we have the choice to aspire.

Faith, like wellness, is dynamic, individual, and universal. Faith, like wellness, exists on a continuum, spanning entire lifetimes. A person's spirit and body are integrated, and to be well one nourishes both. When one chooses faith in God, illness often profits the soul as it forces us to depend on God. Sometimes personal sufferings teach us greater love for others. Problems, such as depression, a broken back, a gluten intolerance, become "spaces" in which one has the opportunity to fervently pray to God. Fr. Roman Braga says, "Suffering is good, not only for Christians, but for everyone, because if you do not suffer, you do not understand anything. [...] After you experience suffering, you understand more—and better—things in this world, much deeper than those who do not experience any suffering."[26]

Recently, a woman from our parish was in a severe auto accident. Upon opening her body and repositioning her organs, doctors counted it a miracle that she had survived. Initially, she couldn't speak and her body was badly broken and bruised. Yet, she signed the cross on a loved one's forearm. Two times before in her life she had been diagnosed with cancer. She had survived. Two months after her accident, she returned to church for an evening service at the beginning of Great Lent. We spoke together in the quiet dim of the banquet hall before others arrived. With a chuckle, she said God didn't want her yet. She said that though her children are grown, God willed for her to be here with us, that there was more for her yet to do in life. Suffering is a gift of perspective. Because of this woman's personal suffering, she felt love for others in pain. That evening in service, I closed my eyes as the words of the Lenten hymns moved through me. I felt the truth of personal suffering as a sure way to empathize with others, and to love them. Because of my own sorrows in earlier times with infertility, marriage, and conversion to the Orthodox Christian faith, I care deeply about others' wellness. In my experiences, wellness is a matter of the body and soul.

---

25 Hymned each Easter in the Orthodox Church.
26 St. Nicholas Orthodox Church, Mentor, OH, parish bulletin, 03 May 2015.

CHAPTER 1
Individualizing Wellness and Saving the Holistic Self

In this book, holistic health is wholeness and holiness, and it is a process of becoming well in the body and spirit. Dn. George Shumaik says, "We can be made whole and spiritually healthy regardless of our physical condition by the grace of God through the Holy Sacraments and in the shelter of His Holy Church. We are called to be holy. We are called to be saints."[27] Physical health is often understood separately from spiritual health, but holistic wellness is a matter of body and spirit because personhood is both the body and the spirit as one whole creation.

Scripture establishes that God created the earth with medicinal properties in herbs and foods.[28] In Genesis, verses show that God provides food for his people: "And God said, 'See, I have given you every herb that yields seed which is upon the face of all the earth, and every tree, whose fruit yields seed; to you it shall be for food.'"[29] Herbs are given for our food and to be eaten: "Thorns also and thistles it shall bring forth for you and you shall eat the herb of the field."[30] Animals were given as food for humankind: "Every moving thing that lives shall be for food for you. I have given you all things, even as the green herbs."[31]

Scripture establishes that God provided medicine for His people through medicinal foods and herbs that abound in nature: "Along the bank of the river, on this side and that, will grow all kinds of trees used for food; their leaves will not wither, and their fruit will not fail. They will bear fruit every month, because their water flows from the sanctuary. Their fruit will be for food, and their leaves for medicine."[32]

Others have plumbed the depths of Scripture to argue for food and herbs as God's intention for our physical wellness, and this is not my primary aim. Some argue that God gave nature and science uses these good gifts to benefit humankind. Certainly, Medicine has brought us comforts: painkillers, life-saving procedures in labor and delivery, and even fertility enhancing medications that enabled me to become pregnant with our first son. Medicine has the capacity to mechanically provide limbs, correct organs, and detect cancers. Countless of us appreciate the benefits of modern medicine; in fact, who could not? What concerns me, however, is the abuse of medication and pharmaceutical

---

27 Shumaik, Dn. George, "Holiness and Wholeness," St. Nicholas Orthodox Church, Mentor, OH, parish bulletin, 03 Oct. 2015.
28 Stanley, Daniel, personal correspondence, 30 Nov. 2015.
29 1:29
30 3:18
31 9:3
32 Ezekiel 47:12

companies that manipulate our need for healing and wellness and profit from our pains.

This costs life.

In the statement issued in 2001 against the use of fetal stem cells, the Holy Synod called Orthodox Christians to consider the meaning and value of life. In faith, I believe that He is, and within the ancient Tradition of Christianity, I seek to understand my life in His. Reflecting on my life in Christ reveals the meaning and purpose of being alive and made in the image and likeness of Jesus Christ. Stories from my life are used throughout this book to serve as illustrations of my responsibility to use the good earth and my created being for life-giving, and this in the face of a world that subtly (and overtly) harms life. I am not a priest or theologian; I am a mother and Christian woman. Using who I am and what I live, I aim to understand the value of life as Jesus Christ teaches us throughout all time in the very lives of saints and sinners alike. It is important to realize that our bodies belong to God.

From the above premise, this chapter focuses on the body and ways that the body can be more well. I have heard it said that a person would only change when the pain of staying the same is worse than the pain of change. As a culture, America is increasingly dependent on drugs and doctors, which haven't made us more well. Many are sick of feeling unwell. This has led me to question what might be done differently concerning health care in order to be more healthy and feel more well.

Experiences with health care over the past decade didn't help me balance hormones, eliminate yeast overgrowth and correct a constantly gurgling gut, or have normal monthly cycles that led to fertility and conception. Changing my diet helped me become more well, and with this change, my lifestyle shifted. I became pregnant within a few months when I changed my diet from high carbohydrates to more protein and calcium. With this dietary change, I also experienced a decrease in anxiety and depression. This may have been a result of feeling better in my bowels because the gut and brain are said to work closely together. At this same time, I trusted God with my body and felt the love and prayers of the Mother of God. These things together made me well.

A decade earlier, I had a yeast overgrowth that upset the hormonal balance of my body and led to various physical problems such as high cholesterol, irritable bowels, anxiety and depression, and infertility. Emotional strain was intense at this time, and I prayed more intensely than ever. I also changed my diet and lifestyle in simple ways. It seemed that healing was a matter of the body and spirit as I prayed. My suffering and healing was experienced in my body and in my spirit through the draw of prayerfulness and the peace that God alone offers each person who chooses to pray to Him.

At the beginning of my journey to becoming more well, I met with a family doctor I had trusted for ten years. She was always open to hear stories of my life, to understand me emotionally and physically. While she, like other doctors, budgeted the valuable minutes we shared, she did so with a keen ability to interpret my emotional and physical needs in symbiotic relationship. Because she had an ability to tie together the workings of my body in relationship to social situations in my life, my over-all well-being was addressed. For example, she listened to my complaints of a sinus infection and also heard the pains of having in-laws move from Russia to the States. At that session, she watched my two small boys bounce around the exam room, and she seemed to understand more than I complained of, as evidenced when she suggested mothering wasn't always easy. With this fuller story in her mind, she counseled me as she was able. She seemed to take seriously my complaints of digestive problems and encouraged me to seek counseling as a way to deal with stress and anxiety. She also referred me to an internist. Interestingly, when I met with the internist, she listened to my narrative only to segue into a number of wasteful tests, going so far as to say that it would be good if I had HIV, which I did not, because then we'd know the root of the "problem." She added that there were many good medications for HIV. I realized then, as I realize even more now, how important it is for doctors to consider the natural balance of patients' bodies and spirits in order to advise them in ways that stops needless run-around and provides more accurate understanding of the patient. Medication was not the answer for me, and it is often not the answer for many other people seeking wellness.

Though I hadn't known what to expect, it seemed to me then that doctors might have inquired more about my diet and lifestyle. Testing my body and comparing results against norms didn't suggest anything specific or telling about my individual condition, though I understood that "norms" were descriptions of common physical conditions. I wrote off my irritable bowel as psychological, though this was really only a result of facing complications in my body caused by other factors. I assumed that I "carried stress in my gut" and that there wasn't much to do to improve conditions. I dismissed my imbalanced hormones, agreeing with doctors who simply said that many women didn't have regulated cycles (even though my menses had actually ceased all together since college). At the time, I wondered why doctors simply provided birth-control pills instead of considering why I hadn't been menstruating. Looking back, I now understand the role of healthy fats in hormone balance. It wasn't a matter of being "too thin," because I was even lighter when my body began cycling normally. Instead, my body needed specific nutrients that it was not getting, a fact that a scale or a diagnostic from the blood laboratory could not reveal, and a fact that was unique to my particular body. I ate well, lots of whole grains, fruits and vegetables; I ate well, according to the rubric of healthy eating in America. Unfortunately, these grains were not agreeing with my system. A discussion about my diet and lifestyle may have led to more helpful suggestions to consuming fewer carbohydrates, etc. Instead, frequent yeast infections had been simply chalked up to a result of a hot summer, though the illness persisted year-round. I was beginning to understand that in current western medical culture, there is a lack of holistic perspective on health. We value objective scientific protocols, even though reading individual patients would lead to more appropriate and less wasteful care in many individuals' lives. Teaching doctors to prescribe medications and see certain diseases replaces honing the necessary skills of discerning individual's ailments in the context of their unique lives. In the long run, many diagnoses are incorrect and patients suffer longer, returning to doctors more often because the sources of their problems haven't been addressed.

Health care, as I have experienced it in current America, tends to approach wellness from the outside in, rather from the inside out. Doctors tend to act on the visible body. Health care providers focus on the body and its physical processes because the predominant medical model since the mid-nineteenth century is "biomedical."[33] In place of the human being, the medical model's focus is on "a human biologic system that can be used to understand normal and abnormal function from gene to phenotype and to provide a basis for preventive or therapeutic intervention in human diseases." Accordingly, "health" constitutes the freedom from disease, pain, or defect. The normal human condition is considered "healthy." The biomedical model generally has four core elements of diagnosing disease and focus is on the physical processes, such as the pathology, the biochemistry, and the physiology of a disease. The role of social factors or individual subjectivity is not significant to the model. The biomedical model is considered the leading modern way for health care professionals to diagnose and treat a condition in most western countries. The fundamental problem is that what we have been saying is healthy is not always, and modern-day food modifications, environmental pollutants, and toxic additives to many foods, medications, and products harm us.

Many people trust what doctors say, and many doctors trust what they are trained to say—until experiences prove otherwise. I recently had an opportunity to observe doctors-in-training at the Cleveland Clinic. Professors in the Humanities led small group discussions on humanism and technology in health care today. Bright young men and women studying to become doctors discussed pressure to master skills and infallibly perform. They communicated the need to separate their human nature from the patient to best perform. We talked about understanding the patient as an individual and feeling empathy. No one argued the need for human care, but a doctor may have more of a responsibility to tend to one's body, a task that could be compromised if the physician is preoccupied with concerns for how the patient feels and thinks. For example, a physician-in-training mentioned a heart surgeon cannot hold one's hand as he operates on the heart. They also argued that certain doctors, like an internist, might care more for patients' individual thoughts and feelings. Some specialists are more likely to explore relationships between a patient's body and mind and the pain(s) for which she presents. For example, oftentimes, Medical Doctors treat one clinical symptom at a time with medication, while those trained in Osteopathic Medicine tend to treat diseases through medication, diet, and lifestyle considerations. For many physicians, the art of their craft is located in objective knowledge and precise execution of their skills, and this doesn't *require* understanding the individual human.

33 "Biomedical Model Definition," *Biomedical Models and Resources: Current Needs and Future Opportunities*, ed. National Research Council, Washington D.C.: National Academic Press, 1988, Chapter 2.

It is valuable to observe a patient carefully to understand their body language because many illnesses have a psychosomatic reality. A doctor-student argued that she couldn't read how people feel, and she doesn't think it is important to do so in her job. Instead, she will read the CT scan accurately. I wondered about reading the patient in order to realize if there's a need for the CT scan. It is a problem to me when doctors are not interested, trained, or personally inclined to understand patients, one human being to another human being, because no matter how skilled one is in diagnosing disease, each body is unique and will manifest illnesses differently. To be holistically well, body and spirit, a human being must be specifically examined with acute attention to subjective details of a patient's body, as well as the objective details of illnesses. Doctors are expected to be confident and to assert medical opinions, and I highly regard a compassionate physician who demonstrates humility and humanity by acknowledging his is a medical "opinion," though based on expertise and disease knowledge. I have found such unassuming doctors are oftentimes the best physicians. Usually, with an attitude of such care, physicians' diagnoses are more accurate. Human interaction in health care is essential, and it seems that today's health care devalues getting to know individual patients and their unique ailments.

Even though diet and lifestyle greatly affect the body, people talk about their "good" or "bad" genes as though one is doomed to be healthy or ill, depending merely on family history. The old adage, "You are what you eat," is very true, but many doctors do not address diet with patients. Instead, the protocol for prevention can be as drastic as when my mother had a hysterectomy so that she wouldn't get ovarian and uterine cancers. Or, when my aunt was told after chemotherapy to eat whatever she liked, it wouldn't change her status with cancer.

In my experience, wellness is a matter of routines that can always improve. A balance of healthy fats, salts, and natural sugars satisfies me. I also feel well with at least six hours of sleep, and moments during the day when I pull away from noise and activity and try to preserve a quiet prayer in my heart. It seems that to be more well as a society, we have to relearn what we thought was good for us. The non-fat diet in the 1990s was unhealthy for many reasons. The body needs healthy fats, and non-fat foods are typically processed, refined, and full of sugar. It is important to eat whole foods that are high in good fats and nutrients and minerals. In fact, vitamins cannot absorb when a body doesn't have essential minerals, which our foods are stripped of (soil is depleted; seeds are modified, for example). Sometimes, simply considering what the ancients ate before microwaves and refined products were available inspires my lunch. Olives, cheese, sweet, dense dates, this can certainly beat a bologna sandwich. I have noticed that what I'm used to eating, I crave. If in a groove of afternoon chocolate-eating, then come three and I'm like a dog sniffing through the freezer. If it's a fasting period, habits of food change, and I've noticed that it is hardest within the first week. After that, new habits form, and I crave coconut oil and almond-butter, for example. Cravings can also signal a nutritional need. A friend mentioned that my desire for cinnamon was a reaction to breastfeeding, fasting, and needing more sugar. It seemed so, after downing a large applesauce with cinnamon. It's important to note that all of our behaviors can change, if we will for them to, like the way we eat, or the way we pray and interact with our children and husband. It takes obedience to get the new routine rolling, but then it rather happens of its own accord: it's just what we do.

Unfortunately, as a culture, we are conditioned to deal with symptom management rather than personal responsibility for diet and lifestyle that contributes to our becoming whole. It isn't entirely our fault. There are endless advertisements for medications on the market, and these drugs promise relief from real pains we suffer. Holistic wellbeing requires the resolve to question why we do what we do, and to be willing to go against the grain, so to speak. It requires that we don't fall for the bias of arguments that simply don't ring true against the reality of our bodies. Holistic wellbeing first and foremost necessitates that one pay careful attention to her behaviors and question what might be better to do. Along with resolve not to make medication one's first option, a person becomes more well with efforts to build the body with balanced (and satisfying) nutrition and moderate movement. If I had to sit still and eat carrot sticks in order to be holistic, I'd take Prozac, too. Eating a salad with beets, eggs, cheese, and a sprinkling of dill-weed, olive oil, and apple cider vinegar, some chips and salty almonds on the side, is really good. I'm not deprived. A walk with the girls to the lake with a few minutes of jumping-jacks in the sunshine, well, this is kind of fun. Each finds her own way. Holistic wellness is accepting the gift of life and finding ways to enjoy living as we build our bodies and feed our spirits. I have spent time sitting in waiting rooms waiting to see a specialist who can unravel the complicated problems of an anxious heart and un-balanced body, and, in my experience, there isn't much that comes from the ten minutes spent with the doctor who reads my vitals and wonders why a healthy young woman is there with him. There are alternatives to medication, and by trying these, we may learn that the body and spirit is able to heal naturally.

In our fallen world, there are real health problems, including diseases and cancers, and there is severe pain. Without a doubt, there are situations that require medical specialists and prescriptions. Thank God that there are highly trained and intelligent physicians that can and do offer life-saving protocols. When my loved ones or I come to such need, I will discern all options to the best of my ability: diet, lifestyle, medication, and various doctors' opinions. Lord have mercy. Suffering is promised in this life, and the wages of sin are death. Life should be recognized as the gift that it is and cared for.

Many people today are asking questions of their doctors and others to find answers to health concerns that are further complicated by prescriptions and their side effects. Additionally, people want answers to why they are ill, which could be explained as variously unbalanced conditions of the whole body. The body as a whole is often not taken into account by health care providers because of a training that does not focus on the holistic person. As doctors routinely prescribe medications and treat patients according to the rubrics of their training, some develop an attitude of intolerance with inquisitive patients, which can exacerbate the problem of patients not trusting their doctors. Many patients get second opinions from others in health care and also seek information on the Internet. Recently, a doctor shook her head and said, "People used to ask a question like, 'Should I get the HPV vaccine?' of an expert, their doctor. Now they're asking that on a blog and getting a reply from someone named Jellyfish. Why aren't we relying on the people who do this for a living?"

It is difficult to know who to trust, and it becomes a matter of turning to our families, friends, and communities, gathering information from sources some consider "quack," and living and learning. With an experience of increased wellness, many people find that these "alternative" sources of information offer more that helps them than a medication with a host of negative side effects. We all wish our doctors would tell us why we are sick, but oftentimes there are no reasonable answers. This leads many to research information on their own. After sifting through alternative news sources, I have learned that many probing individuals have also been gathering scientific evidence and anecdotal observations in order to explain the illnesses they or loved ones suffer. Unfortunately, finding information that counters the government's claims: Federal Drug Administration (FDA), and the United States Centers for Disease Control and Prevention (CDC), turns peoples' attention from health issues to political issues. It also seems to launch people into debates on science versus non-science (as though one alone is true). Science is a dynamic and multifaceted means of explaining life's phenomenon that aims to describe how things work. A person assigns subjective reasoning to further explain why it works as it does and what this means to human beings. "Science" is not entirely objective or unified in these explanations. Unfortunately, in regards to current health care, it is just too obvious, when we look, that pharmaceutical and food corporations are involved in the government's claims on our health.

Our family's journey towards more holistic wellness began when we discovered that our first son had peanut, sugar-snap pea, and shellfish allergies. My son could die from a single ingested peanut, just as six million others[34], or eight percent of children in America today. In 2008, the peanut allergy was up three-fold from 1997, and we continue to see increases in the peanut allergy in westernized countries. In underdeveloped areas of the world such as Africa and Asia, where they do not have westernized health care, peanut allergies are extremely rare. The story is the same for other food allergies: significantly up, though not in places that do not vaccinate as we do. When we met with allergists and I inquired why allergies were more common today, there was no sane answer provided—ever. In a nutshell, the response was: "Allergies just happen; they always have; to which pharmacy should we call in the Epi-pen-jr. and the Albuterol inhaler?" When I conceived my second son, allergists advised that I avoid eating peanut butter and tree-nuts (for cross-contamination) during pregnancy and while breastfeeding. Then, five years later, when pregnant with our third child, doctors said that eating peanut butter did not cause allergies and could even prevent allergies. I was uncomfortable with the

---

34 "Facts and Statistics—Food Allergy Research and Education," http://www.foodallergy.org, Food Allergy Research and Education, Inc., 2015, web, 02 July 2015.

lack of explanation for my son's allergies and the conflicting advice on how to prevent allergies in our growing family. Additionally, I began to realize that doctors did not have all of the answers, nor, in some cases, did they seem to be seeking to explain why children were increasingly suffering with allergies, gut sensitivities, and various developmental delays. They were trained to understand illnesses and diseases, and many separated this understanding from individual patients. As a field, Medicine increasingly seemed to be relying on managing symptoms, rather than finding root-causes of illness and disease. It seemed to me then that many doctors weren't enough concerned with a person being healthy. Unbeknownst to me, my husband began investigating "Jellyfish," and our family began to observe Daddy eating—and smelling—oddly.

He introduced our family to the essential oil of oregano[35] on a summer trip to the Upper Peninsula, MI. My husband ate graham crackers that smelled strongly of oregano, which he'd mixed with nut-butter. He said he'd been researching the health benefits of oregano oil (mixed with a carrier oil such as extra virgin olive oil). At the time, it had smelled gross to our family, but we have learned better ways of using it since the initial graham cracker experiment. We put oregano oil in a medicine bottle, one part essential oil to four parts carrier oil. We take two drops under the tongue daily. Our son's lungs benefited the most. He rarely coughs, no longer has asthma, and is well—without any medication. Oregano oil is very helpful for bronchial ailments, and it is a natural antibiotic with anti-fungal properties. We still and always will have Epi-pens: at school, in his hockey bag, in my purse, and in the kitchen in case he would accidentally ingest peanut, sugar-snap peas, or shellfish. The cost of this medication, with full insurance, is 50.00 for two Epi-pens, and they expire each year. The cost last year for two of the same prescriptions, with the same insurance, was $10.00. Medications that so many children now rely on are increasingly expensive. Pharmaceutical companies are profiting from life-long patrons.

My husband continued bringing strange-to-us-at-the-time packages: colloidal silver water (which we gargle for a sore throat or dab on a cotton ball for a skin irritation), organic vitamins, colloidal minerals (a tablespoon with juice in the morning), and bee-pollen mixed with raw honey. Our family's health was strengthened. I now swear by raw garlic, onions, unrefined, organic coconut oil, and other healthy fats such as avocado, unprocessed, aged cheeses, and even butter. Food helps one maintain a healthy immune system by nourishing the whole body naturally, without potential side effects from medications.

It is helpful to read about topics and talk to professionals, but it is equally important to be mindful of the experiences we have in our bodies. For example, which foods lead to feeling well; which exercises help one's body; and even which prayers make most

---

35 Group, Dr. Edward, "10 Uses for Organic Oregano Oil," http://www.globalhealingcenter.com/natural-health/10-uses-organic-oregano-oil/, Global Healing Center, 21 Jan. 2013, web, 15 April 2015.

sense to a person, all become ways to understand our own bodies and spirits. It is also important to pay attention to our children, particularly after medications. Rather than dismissing their responses, I believe we help our family the most when we listen and watch carefully in order to determine whether a food or activity might be a better choice than a drug that may interact with other systems in the body.

Sometimes, a person has to radically change diet and or lifestyle, with or without medication, to be well. I recently read an interesting article by Andrew Scarborough, "Healing Brain Cancer with a Zero Carb Ketogenic Diet."[36] He shares how he had been on a low fat, high carb diet when he was diagnosed with brain cancer. After failing to improve with chemotherapy and radiation, he began to apply drastic changes in his diet in a desperate attempt to be well. Many doctors told him that his efforts were futile, and that he wouldn't be able to alter his cancer by diet. However, in experimenting with a low-carbohydrate, high-fat diet, he began to improve. At first, he adopted a diet of low sugar fruits and vegetables, lots of heavy whipping cream, coconut milk and oil, nuts, cheese, avocados, etc. He still felt awful, and decided to lower his carbohydrates. He began to improve and feel well as the headaches and seizures reduced. When he again altered his diet to animal fats like butter and tallow and engaged a zero carb carnivorous ketogenic diet, he was even able to stop taking medications as he had almost complete symptom relief. Scarborough argues that this diet is the most efficacious for brain cancer management and improved seizure control.

When a doctor tells a person that they will not live and there is nothing that can be done, then modern medicine reaches its limits. In desperation, some turn to alternative approaches, but diet and lifestyle should not be considered alternative approaches to being well. These should be considered first and foremost before patients are ill, and considerations of changes to diet and lifestyle may help heal one who is ill. Becoming whole begins with our mentality of taking care of the body and spirit. When possible, whole foods and healthful activities should be our line of prevention, rather than surgeries and medications.

Once I learned how easy it was to be more well by changing my diet and using fewer products that contain harmful chemicals, I wanted to learn more and do more on my own, without insurance companies, medications, and doctors referring me to other doctors. Other cultures use foods, herbs, and oils to heal and more naturally balance. For example, food is medicine to Native American, Alaska Native, and Native Hawaiian healers who have a long history of using indigenous, or native, plants for a wide variety of medicinal purposes.[37] Depression in the West is treated with drugs, but food can

36 Scarborough, Andrew, "Healing Brain Cancer with a Zero Carb Ketogenic Diet," http://Zerocarbzen.com/2015/05/31/healing-brain-cancer-with-a-zero-carb-ketogenic-diet-by-andrew-scarborough/, blog, 31 May 2015, web, 15 June 2015.
37 "Medicine Ways: Traditional Healers and Healing," https://www.nlm.nih.gov/nativevoices/exhibition/healing-ways/medicine-ways/healing-plants.html *Native*

improve brain chemistry. For example, cashews are rich in tryptophan, which the body converts to serotonin, and two handfuls decrease depression and help sleep. The nut includes minerals like copper and magnesium and is cheaper than Prozac, which studies have linked to suicidal tendencies.[38]

Other cultures use herbs because they taste good and are healthful[39], and I find that it is easy and delicious to add herbs to all sorts of foods that are popular in America— from burgers to pizza to baked potatoes, a little dill weed, oregano, basil, and parsley is a good addition. My mother-in-law always sets out fresh dill and cilantro, to sprinkle on everything from tomato and cucumber salads to rice and fried meats. I had never tasted fresh tarragon and rosemary on mashed potatoes and salmon, but when I did, the flavor was amazing. There are many health benefits of fresh herbs. For example, tarragon is very good for the female reproductive organs and prevents cancers. Rosemary and oregano helps with inflammation and counters arthritis. Dill is high in calcium, magnesium, and many other nutrients. Parsley helps prevent breast cancer. A friend blends cilantro and cucumber and blueberry smoothies because of the benefits to the liver and kidneys, which work to detox the body of heavy metals.

In my experiences with conception, pregnancy, and postpartum health care, holistic health is up to the individual patient. Some doctors are narrowly concerned with the facts; pregnant: when was your last period; after birth: do you have pain, is the baby latching on, or do you want formula; postpartum: is the baby gaining weight? Simple concerns for a woman's holistic wellness might be addressed with such inquiries as what are you eating and how can you incorporate more whole, nutrient-rich foods into your diet? What exercise can you and the baby engage? A doctor might question a person's psychological and physical wellbeing, beyond asking if a new mom is depressed, by asking: How are you handling stress and what creative outlets to you have for work and adult interaction? Understandably, one's OBGYN cannot care for all of a woman's needs, and maybe some do discuss real concerns with women they've built a relationship with through her pregnancy and birth. I encourage even more recognition of patients' foundational body-spirit composition. Appreciation of personhood would revolutionize our culture and its health care by relating physical and spiritual health and fostering simple ways for individuals to understand wellness.

A midwife led me through my fourth pregnancy and delivery. I had hoped for a more "natural" experience, and I communicated this desire. My pregnancies were without complications, and I didn't want procedures that were unnecessary for me. While she was caring and compassionate, very little was different from having had doctors, all of

Peoples' Concepts of Health and Illness: Native Voices, U.S. National Library of Medicine, 2015, web, 07 July 2015.
38 Saul, Dr. Andrew, "Prozac Alternatives," http://www.doctoryourself.com/prozac.html, DoctorYourself.com, 15 Mar 2014, web, 10 May 2015.
39 Nearing, Margaret "Five Benefits of Fresh Herbs," http://www.besthealthmag.ca/best-eats/nutrition/5-health-benefits-of-fresh-herbs, 2015, *Best Health Magazine*, web, 02 July 2015.

the same tests and drugs were administered—as they routinely are for patients my age, race, and in similar "normal" condition. I was nauseous in the beginning of my pregnancy, and my mid-wife prescribed Zofran. I became constipated after one pill, which is another natural issue in early pregnancy, and the suffering was great in a new way. After taking my prescription and talking with a friend, she mentioned that the FDA approved a drug for nausea in pregnancy, Diclegis, with the highest safety rating, though this drug had been pulled from the market 30 years ago. Even scarier, I now understand that Zofran recently caused severe birth defects, including cleft lip and palate. Just because medications are available and considered safe, in many cases one is better off not to take it. In my experience, coping with the body's natural pains through food and herbs, exercise, and healthful drinks spares me the unpleasant side effects and risks that may occur with medication.

As mothers, being well is necessary so that we can care for our families. Dr. Oscar Serrallach[40], a family practitioner in rural Australia who works at a clinic to treat women for post-natal depletion, says that many mothers (up to 50 %) are depleted of vital nutrients before conception and even ten years after having a child. He says that women fail "hormonally, nutritionally, and emotionally—to get back on their feet after the baby comes." Mothers become "tired and wired" because of the natural demands and changes to mothers' bodies that are already depleted leading up to pregnancy. The placenta is designed to feed the baby and the mother, and 60 % of the placenta goes to the developing baby's brain. To develop a healthy placenta and to balance and rebalance hormones, one needs a nutrient-rich diet, which we are not getting in our foods (because they are grown in less nutrient-rich soil and we eat too many processed foods and not enough organic whole foods). Serrallach argues that with relatively balanced nutrients and minerals, the mother and baby interactively produce hormones that help the child to be born and develop after birth. Breastfeeding continues through a hormonally charged exchange between the baby and mother. He argues that our culture fails to respect nature: "[T]he further we drift away from this in terms of interventions such as caesarian surgery, and opting not to breastfeed, the more we can expect the 'cascade-like' flow of 'compromises' in the postpartum period and beyond, for mother and baby." Dr. Serrallach continues, saying that a woman's brain shrinks five percent during pregnancy, but that the role of the placenta is to re-program the brain to intuit the needs of the infant: if the baby is cold, hungry, ill, etc. When a woman is tired and spent, physically and emotionally, she is less able to care for her children.

Many assume women suffer baby-blues in the first four months postpartum, but Serrallach argues that women are depleted four to seven years after birth. Symptoms of depletion include fatigue and exhaustion, tired on waking, falling asleep unintentionally, hyper-vigilance (feeling tired and wired), sense of guilt and shame as a mother and loss of self-esteem (also feeling isolated and apprehensive about normal things like leaving

---

40 Serrallach, Dr. Oscar, "Postnatal Depletion—Even 10 Years Later," http://goop.com/postnatal-depletion-even-10-years-later/, 5 May 2015, web, 10 July 2015.

the house), no time for one's self, fog-brain, and loss of libido. Interestingly, many of these symptoms are characteristic of depression and anxiety.

Too often today, normal disequilibrium of the body and spirit is classified as illness. Others and I have complained of such postpartum experiences. With my first son, I especially dealt with such depletion and hadn't understood then how much diet and lifestyle affect the body. With intense stress in my life at the time, I hadn't realized what was happening to my body. I trusted well-meaning doctors who had been trained to treat ailments, and I continued on a run-around for answers that never came from the doctors. Even in times when I hadn't felt well, medication was not something I felt that I needed or wanted. I had seen how depression and anxiety worsened over time with the use of pharmaceuticals, and I preferred to run. Of course, each one is different, and I'm not saying that all who are depressed and anxious run and forgo medication. However, natural ways of changing brain chemistry and increasing the body's strength and stamina will directly help one's psychological well-being.

In some cases, medicine for the body and mind saves lives. In other situations, medication becomes a crutch, and then a dependence and people do not moderate and balance their own bodies, as they might otherwise have learned to do. In my life, a healthful diet, active lifestyle, and reflective mind-set foster wellness. Rather than taking medication for mental "illnesses," it seems to me that many times we just need to get a bit more of a grip on how we are living. Other times, however, we are living through a trauma and may need more intervention to help us through. In cases much rarer than is commonly assumed today, one is mentally ill and requires medication. I think it is best when diet and lifestyle is always considered alongside medication.

Today, many psychological problems are blamed on various factors other than diet and lifestyle. People I love have taken medication for manic depression, and I have witnessed how years of taking prescription drugs keeps one dependent on doctors and health care. Pain is the body's natural mechanism to alert one to the need for balance. In some cases, dulling pain provides an out for escaping the need to address deeper issues related to the body and soul. Some new research even suggests that depression can be caused by inflammation in the brain.[41] Depression can often be a result of physical and spiritual disquiet that is impossible to avoid in this life. Sometimes, life seems too hard: a son leaves for college; one is diagnosed with cancer, a child's experience with chemotherapy. The body and spirit can seem deflated. We must weep, have mercy on our own fallen and humble human condition, and take help that may indeed free us from our struggles enough to see how to pick up our spirits and endure our bodies once again. There is no place for guilt when we have a need for medication. The root of the failure in health care today is the over-reliance on medication, but not the use of it all

41 McNamee, David, "Severe depression linked with inflammation in the brain," http://www.medicalnewstoday.com/articles/288715.php, *Medical News Today*, 29 Jan. 2015, web, 12 June 2015.

together.

Life's journey is long and hard, and feeling stable is fleeting because once we get to a "place," we immediately begin another journey. For example, this past year, I gave birth, our family moved, and I completed a PhD in Composition and Rhetoric. It was all said and done by the end of summer, and I stood on our deck looking out at the night. There was a feeling of contrast between the constancy of day that always fell to night and the unknowns of my personal life. The breeze brushed against my face, and in a moment, I was still, calm, and happy. The reality of faith in this life seemed to me than a choice to believe that good would be, just as the day would set to night. Faith shifts my will according to confidence in God, and imparts gratitude that weaves in and out of my fallen perspective on all things. In stabilizing moments, I feel compassion for others, God, and myself. When unsettled, memory can draw me back to faith. The feelings have to be endured, but emotions are always passing. Truth is living with faith in what is good and aspiring to wholeness.

Medication is like most consumer products: over-done, over-marketed, and over-relied upon. My confidence is shaken in "princes of men," in whom there is no salvation, as we sing in Liturgy. Doctors are knowledgeable, but they are not God. It is important to listen to experts and take the good that is offered with a discerning mind. Wellness is complex, and rather than depend on others to fix every whim that pains us, we may become more responsible for the interconnectedness of the body and spirit and practice moderation with commonsense that doesn't require an MD or a PhD. It takes work to care for our bodies, but once the ball gets rolling, maintaining wellness is easier than living unwell. Discernment is difficult in consumeristic western culture. My friend and mentor, as well as brilliant psychologist and scholar, Dn. Stephen Muse mentioned that to keep the "wheel going" the media "manufactures consent" and changes the sobriety of the "spiritual immune system." Indeed, it is a challenge to see clearly, but when our bodies and spirits are ill, we have a unique opportunity to re-evaluate things because we feel a great need to.

Christians preserve the sanctity of life, no matter what, believing by faith that God understands what we cannot at a given point in time—perhaps ever. My husband mentioned an etymology of the word "understand" comes from builders who stood under their project looking up in order to better see how to proceed. Life experiences, knowledge learned, and reflection on personal experiences, provide opportunities for human beings to understand many things. Personal experiences lead me deeper into faith in God, and with faith in Him, I seek knowledge and understanding. My efforts are with faith in God, the Giver of Life, Who alone understands the full picture, and to whom I pray for help. I cannot understand the dynamism of the body and spirit, but I can respect it. In addition, if I do, then I can appreciate that I have a soul and body, and my life is a gift from God.

One very popular approach today to all sorts of issues, particularly with the body, is that everyone has an opinion and a right to their own opinion. Truth is made out to be relative, and discussions are often battles of ideas. It is better when we seek Truth and are open to changing our minds, accepting that we do not know everything already. Information should actually inform us, and we shouldn't just work out an argument against it.

The following chapter discusses research on vaccination. I ask you to consider this chapter with the understanding that the practice of vaccination has arisen because of our current medical paradigm, as discussed in this chapter. My opinion on vaccines is that they are ugly and evil. What matters most are the following facts (make your own opinions): vaccines are produced using fetal stem cells from aborted babies. The Orthodox Church states that under no circumstance should Orthodox Christians use fetal stem cells from aborted babies. There are harmful preservatives and antigens in vaccines that are necessary for the vaccine to be produced. These ingredients harm one's body. Sometimes the body reacts right away to vaccines, and other times the harm is dormant until a later time in one's life. One example of bodily harm that can and does occur from vaccination is sterilization. Many are infertile today. These are facts.

No one that I know began with a position against vaccination. It was after harm, usually to one's child, that minds changed. Then lifestyles. A fight for life is needed in this world. Life situations should be reflected upon, and learned from. We are made better through this approach to living. In a discussion concerning vaccination, a friend said that both sides always stand firm. I replied that this should not be so. We must be open to changing our minds, if experiences with wellness do not align with the practices of our health care. We should consider what we believe and think, feel and understand, seeking the truth with reverence for the fact that Truth will always be fuller than it is possible to understand.

The best way to navigate faith and wellness in this lifetime is to allow experiences and knowledge to inform my choices, and through each step along the way seek Wisdom through prayer. I believe that to individualize wellness and save the holistic self, each of us should pay careful attention to our own bodies and the bodies of our children, parents, and all others we care for. When possible, it is better to live naturally balanced with foods and activities that help us to be well and to limit medications. There is no dietary change or lifestyle enhancement that can produce immortality. Living to eat, drink, and be merry is sad because life is more. Life has purpose and meaning. It is sacred. With respect for our own bodies and souls, and others', we can love life and increase good in the world.

CHAPTER 2
Preserving Life and Nurturing Natural Immunity

*Science can explain away common sense. Pride can refuse to
be wrong, and faith can outright reject eugenics.*

A person is well through diet, lifestyle, and basic hygiene. The history of vaccines, beginning with smallpox in the 1800s, clearly shows that communities are healthier without vaccines and without filth. Though it may sound strange to add vaccines to filth, as the cause of disease, but this is so.[42] Vaccines cannot create stronger health. This is a fact: each vaccine necessarily includes animal and or human cells and harmful adjuvants, and the adjuvants themselves are necessary to produce the antigen response argued as the reason for the success of vaccination. There is absolutely no safe and effective vaccine based on the necessary ingredients in each vaccine. Likewise, it is impossible to produce an ethical vaccine because of the very ingredients included in their formulation.

I am not a scientist and do not speak of vaccination as a scientist, though I quote many who are in the course of this argument. I have a message that scientists I know and love, even some with whom I share Christianity, seem unable and or unwilling to understand. My explanation of cells, DNA, and protein will not include the knowledge base of a scientist, and this is not my book's intent: I do not aim to convince readers of my grasp of the human body's functions. Rather, with faith in the Giver of Life, I tremble at the mystery of the body—its intricate systems and its phenomenal ability to heal and be well, when one works with nature. With reverence for the sanctity of life, I wish to share what my heart intuits, as well as my mind understands to the degree that I am able. I seek Truth with my whole self, openly confessing that I cannot understand everything. A medical doctor near and dear to me told me that because I admittedly do not understand science (as a medical doctor would), it would be difficult to persuade her. On the flip side, I argue my perspective allows me to consider scientific explanations that are not commonly held in allopathic medicine. With common sense, we can both see that kids today are ill, but as she explains it as a result of things such as I-pods, poor eating habits, and lacking family care, I understand these negative effects on children are in addition to the primary problem of vaccination. Certainly, I am not alone. Those who have any interest in understanding why and how vaccines harm us should view three powerful websites chock-full of scientific studies, testimonials, and expertise: www.educate4theinjured.org, https://cogforlife.org, and www.learntherisk.org.

As a scholar of argument and a writer of stories, I observe humanity—the ways people interact, react, feel, think, and use language. My interest the past decade, based

---

42 Humphries, Dr. Suzanne, Roman Bystrianyk, *Dissolving Illusions: Disease, Vaccines, and the Forgotten History*, http://www.dissolvingillusions.com, book summary, web, 26 Jan. 2016.

on my own health conditions and my scholarship in biomedical humanities, has led me deeper into the meaning of holistic wellness. My efforts here include careful observation of life and an account of science from those who argue from a shared position against vaccination. Medical doctors, scholars, and scientists sacrifice deserved respect in their professions when they conclude, after a professional catalyst leads them to look again, that the obvious ills of vaccination cannot be denied. I praise God that such individuals stand strong and explain vaccination from their scientific understanding. May many others use their expertise and help our world understand.

One of the most important issues to me all the way through my journey to understand vaccination continues to be the use of fetal stem cells. Fetal stem cells are used in the production of vaccines. The viruses of 23 vaccines were cultured in the organs of aborted babies. Many fetuses were tried but failed to "work" before the selection of the cell line from the aborted fetus. A friend likened stem cells in vaccines to a tea bag in a cup of hot water. Though the tealeaves do not remain in the mug, the tea includes particles from the leaves. The vaccine includes human DNA from fetal stem cells in which the virus was cultured.

From my research, personal experiences, and social observations, I have come to regard vaccines harmful and as an assault on the sanctity of life. To be clear, fetal stem cells are used in the production of vaccines, though this is not the only reason that vaccines assault life. By injecting foreign human and animal DNA into one's deep muscle tissue (which can and does enter one's bloodstream), one's vitality is threatened, and this harms life. Today, there is a corporate mechanism in place: the abortion and medical industries together with the pharmaceutical companies claim that abortion is a good and necessary reality to save lives through vaccines. Last year a baby was aborted every minute and a half. It becomes like paddling up-river to unravel how things could have gone so wrong to a society unwilling to believe that history is repeating itself. It is understandable that people would doubt, the truth concerning vaccines was covered up from the beginning by belief in a miracle tonic (vaccine), even though statistics demonstrate that communicable diseases were over 90 percent eradicated before vaccines (and antibiotics) were used. You needn't take my word for it. The facts are included in many accounts, such as meticulously compiled in Dr. Humphries' *Dissolving Illusions*.

The truth is that vaccines do not save lives, and many are harmed in small and great ways by vaccines. This has been the case, and known by many scientists and doctors, not to mention parents, since the 1800s, when vaccines were introduced, and through to present times. Individuals are not informed of health conditions caused by vaccines. Unbelievably, people who are pregnant and or have immune-suppressed conditions are rarely offered thimerosal-free vaccines, such as for the flu, even though the toxic preservative has been proven very hazardous for these individuals' health. The sanctity of others' lives is also risked through vaccination. In an over-fifty page report, Barbara Fisher comprehensively presents data to demonstrate, "The Emerging Risks of Live Virus and Virus Vectored Vaccines: Vaccine Strain Virus Infection, Shedding, and Transmission: A Referenced Report from the National Vaccine Information Center."[43] For example, the combination DTaP vaccine (containing diphtheria, tetanus, and pertussis antigens) is causing pertussis in adolescents and infants with older siblings.[44] The best defense against pertussis is a natural source of vitamin C, free of harmful additives and non-synthetic (not ascorbic acid). Yet this information is not communicated to individuals seeking health care, and I believe withholding such important information is also a direct assault on the sanctity of life. Harm has been proven to occur after vaccination, and yet the United States government does not hold pharmaceutical companies liable. In fact, the making of "ethical" vaccines is currently blocked, according to Fr. Baldwin. Aborting babies and harming others has some advantage to those who make money taking care of health needs. Bottom line: vaccines harm and hinder wellness. It is safer to risk the illnesses that we are vaccinated against than it is to receive current vaccinations.[45] Children are suffering.

Today's children receive 29 times the amount of vaccines as those born 30 years before—most of which are given when in early childhood. Before a child is five today, the CDC recommends 51 vaccines, two in utero (DTaP and flu). Unbelievably, the influenza vaccine has never been tested on pregnant women (though it is recommended anyways). In 2009-10, fetal deaths reported to the Vaccine Adverse Event Reporting System (VAERS) increased by 4,250% with the recommendation that pregnant women get the flu shot. It seems to many parents that there really aren't that many more vaccines, but the multiple vaccines administered in one shot mask this. The harm is magnified in such vaccinations, as parents with vaccine-injured children will attest, and the fact is that safety studies are lax and insufficient to determine safety and efficacy. The irony of giving a newborn a vaccination for hepatitis B, even when the mother is tested and negative is ludicrous. It is even worse considering the amount of aluminum (250mcg) in this vaccine is 10 times the FDA's "safe" amount (25mcg). Such abuse must be stopped.

The silencing of voices speaking out is astonishing. For example, Jasmine Yuzwak[46] from "Green Med" writes of the shocking & damming interview regarding vaccine injury with Dr. Judy Mikovits, a PhD in Biochemistry, and a cellular and molecular biologist with over 30 years of scientific expertise. In 2011 when she made a horrifying discovery that

43 Fisher, Barbara, "The Emerging Risks of Live Virus and Virus Vectored Vaccines: Vaccine Strain Virus Infection, Shedding, and Transmission: A Referenced Report from the National Vaccine Information Center," http://www.nvic.org/CMSTemplates/NVIC/pdf/Live-Virus-Vaccines-and-Vaccine-Shedding.pdf, National Vaccine Information Center, 2014, web, 01 Sept. 2015.
44 Hammond, Jeremy, "The Ugly Untold Truth About the Pertussis Vaccine," http://www.jeremyrhammond.com/2015/09/14/the-ugly-untold-truth-about-the-pertussis-vaccine/, *Foreign Policy Journal*, 14 Sept. 2015, web, 30 Sept. 2015.
45 Tietje, Kate, "Which is Safer: Vaccines or Illnesses?," http://www.modernalternativemomma.com/2014/10/03/safer-vaccines-illnesses/, *Modern Alternative Momma*, 2015, web, 08 Oct. 2015.
46 Yuswak, Jasmine, "Interview with Dr. Judy Mikovits, PhD," http://vimeo.com/146831570, 22 Nov. 2015.

was contaminating all vaccinations, she presented her data to government officials and was threatened and told to destroy all her data. When she did not, she was jailed, her career systematically destroyed, and a gag order put in place for four years. If she spoke out, she would be thrown back in jail. Recently, the gag order lifted, and she spoke about how autism is associated with vaccines, cancers, chronic fatigue syndrome, Alzheimer's, autoimmune diseases, allergies and more. She discusses how the cocktail of vaccinations pumped into babies mutate to develop months and years later into new viruses, cancers and diseases, some they don't even know about yet. She explains how the viruses injected through vaccines tear open our DNA and insert their own DNA to mutate our genetic makeup and be passed on generation after generation. She has been threatened with a suicide murder cover up, but chose to expose what she knows.

One who is open-minded to consider why a person would be anti-vaccine will easily realize a fuller picture. Those who consider the wealth of current information on vaccination, some of which I cover in what follows, with a mind and heart seeking truth, will see a pressing need to become as personally informed as possible about wellness. Today's western health care is failing us in two main ways: vaccines and over-medication. We owe it to ourselves and our children to turn towards living more whole and holy lives.

The vaccination program in the United States gained momentum at the same time as the biomedical model of health care in the mid-1900s. Bodies were acted upon, and the effects were compartmentalized. Today, there are many reasons why vaccination is barbaric, and why it always has been. To begin with, I believe that injecting aborted fetal stem cells and foreign human DNA into another human being is horrific to anyone with a conscience. It is deplorable, though understandable, that as a culture we believe in vaccines as a way to be free of disease. For the following reasons, I will not vaccinate my children or myself in the future: vaccines have never lessened disease but increased it; fetal stem cells are used; toxic adjuvants are included in vaccines, and these are necessary to cause the antigen effect (which means they cannot be removed from the vaccine formulation). Vaccination increases rates of disease, the immune system is weakened and vaccination has never produced "herd immunity." Diseases do not manifest in societies where water is clean and people are not living in filth because of sewer systems and basic hygiene practices.

As a mother, I see that the obvious bias in favor of vaccination fails against the crisis of health among children today in the U.S. As a Christian, I aim to understand vaccine harm in light of my faith in God who provides life and to whom I am indebted to preserve life entrusted to me, my own and the children given to me. Understanding vaccine harm also concerns me as a friend, neighbor, and simply a member of society who believes in the right to health. I'm not a medical doctor or scientist, though I borrow scientific research from those who are[47] in what follows. Using scientific research that presents facts on vaccine harm, as well as stories of my life and others' lives, I share a fleshed-out picture that cannot be dismissed as a "political issue" by those who value the sanctity of life.

The following is my attempt to explain why the current vaccination program in the States is unacceptable, and it is my hope that the many mothers and fathers who care with all of their hearts for the wellbeing of their children will choose not to follow their well-meaning, though (in many cases) uniformed pediatricians. Unfortunately, accepting this message means that one is willing to consider a very unbelievable reality: pharmaceutical companies provide funding for institutions of higher learning, the United States government, and our media. A lot of money. There are increasing conflicts of interest in medical education[48], and pharmaceutical companies are primarily concerned with profit, not health.

Since the mid-twentieth century, false confidence in vaccines has led to a theory of wellness that has increasingly made us ill. Now, it is past the point of denying when we look at children riddled with disorders from severe food allergies to brain damage. Some argue, I / my child were vaccinated and are fine. Unfortunately, as Michael Skinner argues[49], toxins that affect an individual may be passed on to one's offspring. While the toxins in our vaccines may not have visibly caused a vaccinated person immediate damage, it is likely that the accumulation of toxins from the outlandish quantity of 73 currently recommended vaccinations (in addition to other toxic influences from our food and environment) will lead to less viable children and grandchildren. I will not vaccinate because it slams against my belief in the sanctity of life, both in living whole and living holy. Acquiring knowledge of vaccination became a spiritual journey with prayer and faith, and it was eye opening to learn of facts that challenged paradigms that I had once accepted.

I was in the back of our parish one Sunday morning, among six or so other mothers and fathers. I know these parents, and they love their children. They bring them to church for the experience of seeking Truth in God. They profess faith in Christ, and as Christians support the sanctity of life. It pained me to think that many of them do not realize that vaccines include aborted fetal stem cells. If a person is pro-life, then they should not vaccinate. It was also troubling to think of the risks they may unknowingly place upon their children through vaccinations.

---

47 Edwards, Joel, "Doctors Against Vaccines—These physicians actually did the research," http://www.naturalnews.com/051421_vaccination_research.html, 04 Oct. 2015, web, 04 Oct. 2015.
48 *Institute of Medicine (US) Committee on Conflict of Interest in Medical Research, Education, and Practice*; Lo B, Field MJ, editors. Washington (DC): National Academies Press (US); 2009. 26 Feb. 2016, web, www.ncbi.nlm.nih.gov/books/NBK22945/.
49 Interlandi, Jeneen, "The Toxins that Affected your Great-Grandparents Could be in Your Genes," *Smithsonian*, http://www.smithsonianmag.com/innovation/the-toxins-that-affected-your-great-grandparents-could-be-in-your-genes-180947644/, Dec. 2013, web, 10 Nov. 2015.

I fear that we are being destroyed from the inside out. Our bodies are harmed by too many medications with vile side effects, and our communities are rife with tensions between accepted practices and knowledge and challenges to these health care norms. Natural health practitioner and enthusiast, Courtney Charles, argues that since the first vaccine, 21 vaccines currently include aborted fetal stem cells, this number is now 23 and rising and there are many more vaccines being created using aborted fetuses. She continues that since the first vaccine there has been nothing but harm from vaccination. After studying the evidence from many other sources, I agree very much with her claims and appreciate her passionate narrative from a Christian perspective.[50]

Mainstream news (such as ABC News) argues that fetal tissue used in vaccines is over 50 years old, and that there may be a "billionth of a gram" in a given vaccine, as much as would be on fruits and vegetables.[51] Like most of the mainstream media coverage on vaccines, this is not the full story, nor is the reason for objection given, according to one who values the sanctity of life. Back in 2010, a pro-life group, Vaccine Awareness of North Florida, provided the "tip of the ice-burg" in a discussion on the assault of life concerning vaccines and fetal stem cells.[52] They argued then that for over thirty years pharmaceutical companies have been quietly producing vaccines using remains of aborted babies. This had been hidden for decades, and now it is "covered up" with claims to minuscule amounts of fetal cells in the vaccine. When pro-life publications revealed the truth, many doctors and parents were shocked. While some media outlets (such as ABC News, and the like) have continued down-playing the issue, the history of using aborted fetuses for research and development of vaccines began in 1964, continues still, and includes an undisclosed number of abortions. I recently wept while watching a video of an abortion in which a twenty-week old fetus has its legs and arms pulled off, intestines drawn out, and once the skull is left alone in the mother's womb, it is smashed and its parts taken piece at a time. Many women would not choose to abort if they saw this. During a rubella outbreak, some doctors advised woman to have abortions for fear of birth defects. Researchers working alongside doctors collected fetal tissue, and the 27th baby's kidneys were used, among "numerous other abortions." 80 elective abortions were performed in the production of the rubella vaccine alone. The practice of encouraging abortions so that fetal tissue may be used in the development of vaccines (and other pharmaceuticals) during a time when a woman is very vulnerable is unacceptable. However, we are accepting it, and this attitude threatens the realization of life as a sacred gift. Such disregard threatens our entire world. Because the pharmaceutical industry perceives public acceptance of the current vaccines, they continue to utilize both existing and new aborted fetal sources for vaccine development.

---

50   Charles, Courtney, "Do Vaccines Violate the Christian Faith?," http://www.alabasterliving.com/blog/do-vaccines-violate-the-christian-faith, personal blog, 16 May 2015, web, 07 July 2015.
51   Neporent, Liz, "What Aborted Fetuses Have to Do With Vaccines – ABC News," http://abcnews.go.com/health/aborted-fetuses-vaccines/story?id=29005539, *ABC News – Breaking US & World News (ABC Digital)*, 17 Feb. 2015, web, 18 May 2015.
52   "K.N.O.W. Vaccines," http://www.know-vaccines.org/, Vaccine Awareness of North Florida, 2010, web, 01 June 2015.

The latest is a new fetal cell line, PER C6, created by Dutch pharmaceutical, Crucell, NV. This cell line uses the retinal tissue of an 18-week gestation baby, created specifically for vaccine development.

A Choice — And A Moral Duty!

Similar to adult stem cell therapies, which are viable alternatives to using destroyed human embryos, some argue that vaccines can be made using ethical sources. Instead, the present tainted vaccines have been used to justify further immoral research. In August 2001, President Bush rationalized funding embryonic stem cell research by using the chickenpox vaccine as a precedent, since the embryos, like the aborted babies, had already been destroyed. However, in both cases, human beings were intentionally and callously slaughtered for research purposes. Unless the public refuses to tolerate this exploitation of our unborn, it will only worsen.

The use of stem cells from aborted fetuses is involved in most vaccines.[53] Planned Parenthood is selling aborted fetuses to pharmaceutical companies, harvesting organs of these tiny human beings even as hearts beat.[54] As a friend said, "How could God bless that?"

New aborted fetal cell lines are in development, and I do not believe that God will bless the effects of vaccines for which these children are sacrificed. In a report from September 9, 2015, from *Children of God for Life*,[55] the following was stated:

Due to dwindling capacity for existing aborted fetal cell lines to self-replicate, scientists in China have developed a new aborted fetal cell line, WALVAX 2 that will be used for viral vaccine production. The existing cell lines, MRC-5 and WI-38 are currently used in MMR, Varicella, Hepatitis-A, Shingles, some rabies and some polio vaccines. WALVAX 2 was taken from the lung tissue of a 3-month gestation female who was ultimately selected from among nine aborted babies. The scientists noted how they followed specific guidelines to mimic WI-38 and MRC-5 in selecting the aborted babies, ranging from 2-4 months gestation. They further noted how they induced labor using a 'water bag' abortion to shorten the delivery time and prevent the death of the fetus to ensure live intact organs, which were immediately sent to the labs for cell preparation.

53 *Children of God for Life*, https://cogforlife.org, 2015, web, 15 Mar. 2015.
54 "Aborted Babies Were Born Alive Before Organ Harvesting," www.edgytruth.com/2015/07/31/aborted-babies-were-born-alive-before-organ-harvesting/, 31 July 2015, web, 1 Aug. 2015.
55 "New Aborted Fetal Cell Line Emerges for Vaccine Production," https://www.lifesitenews.com/opinion/new-aborted-fetal-cell-line-emerges-for-vaccine-production, Opinion, *LifeSite*, 09 Sept. 2015, web, 02 Feb. 2016.

According to the studies published earlier this year in the NIH Pub Med, scientists noted that WALVAX-2 cells replicated more rapidly than MRC-5 cells, attained greater population doubling and performed better or equal to the existing cell lines for culturing viruses.

In 1964 Leonard Hayflick introduced what is known as the "Hayflick limit" – how all normal cells have a finite lifespan and limited capacity to replicate before going into senescence and eventually become unstable and form tumors. (L. Hayflick, The Limited In Vitro Lifetime of Human Diploid Cell Strains, Experimental Cell Research, Vol 37, 1964). Attempts to immortalize these cells to extend their lifespan have likewise introduced problems with tumor formations, as in aborted fetal cell line PER C6, introduced into the US in 2001.
Such seems to be the case with the introduction of WALVAX 2 to replace Hayflick's WI-38 and Medical Research Council's MRC-5. Instead of choosing from several, WHO and FDA approved moral cell lines to replace them, they are using a new aborted fetal source.

'This is exactly what we have been saying for years,' stated Debi Vinnedge, Executive Director for Children of God for Life, an organization that has been monitoring the use of aborted fetal materials in vaccines and other consumer products. 'The pharmaceutical industry is not going to change their use of aborted fetal cells when they have tacit approval from our moral and medical leaders.'

For decades both the pharmaceutical companies and even some ethicists have insisted that the abortions to produce the cell lines used in vaccines were not done with that intention, that it was only a couple of abortions from the past, and that no further abortions would be needed 'now or in the future' to produce vaccines.

'This may be the biggest lie ever told to the American public and the world at large,' said Mrs. Vinnedge. 'Not only have there been hundreds of abortions directly involved with vaccine research—specifically for that purpose where they altered abortion methods to obtain intact fetal organs—but we are now seeing more and more abortions for fetal research and new cell lines emerging for viral vaccine cultivation.'

Few of us were ever told that our children's vaccines were cultured on fetal stem cells from aborted fetuses. Instead, we are simply advised to get our flu shots when pregnant—never, ever warned that the flu shot was shown to increase miscarriage by over 4,000% from 1990-2009[56]. Until 2015-2016, fetal stem cells were also used in the development of the flu shot.[57] When I asked if getting the shot was safe in pregnancy, I was assured that it was completely safe and necessary, so that I wouldn't get the flu. Unbeknownst to me at the time, the flu shot does not protect against the flu[58] and has harmful adjuvants that should never be injected into a pregnant woman. The mercury, thimerosal, in the flu shot can travel to the central nervous system and it is stored in fat cells. Thimerosal is a recognized neurotoxin, and the vaccine industry has argued that the preservative is being phased out of vaccines; however, this is not true. Lord Joel from the Vaccine Resistance Movement claims:

> Contrary to all the Vaccine Industry rhetoric & double-speak we're forced to swallow as a community of a unilateral plan to completely phase-out its use, the truth reveals that thimerosal mercury is still being added, by design, 'ostensibly' as a sterilant/preservative, in numerous vaccines on the standard immunization schedule.

> Quantities/traces of thimerosal (average 25-75 µg/micrograms) are currently found in the following vaccines:
> a. Influenza vaccine (multi-dose) – 'Afluria,' 'Fluzone,' 'Fluvirin, 'FluLaval'
> b. Hepatitis B vaccine – 'Engerix,' 'Twinrix'
> c. Diphtheria, tetanus, pertussis vaccine (series) – 'Tripedia'
> d. Haemophilus influenzae type b vaccine (multi-dose vials) – 'ActHIB®'
> e. Meningococcal polysaccharide vaccine – 'Menomune'
> f. Measles, mumps, rubella vaccine – 'M-M-R II'
> g. Tetanus toxoid vaccine – no trade name/ manufactured by Sanofi Pasteur[59]

Thimerosal is one of the most dangerous substances for a human being and should never be given to a pregnant woman, according to Dr. Suzanne Humphries.[60] Though there are available flu vaccines that do not contain thimerosal, most do, and in amounts above federal safety guidelines. One has to ask their health care provider for the flu shot

---

56 England, Christina, "4,250% Increase in Fetal Deaths Reported to VAERS After Flu Shot Given to Pregnant Women," https://vactruth.com/2012/11/23/flu-shot-spikes-fetal-death/, Vactruth, 23 Nov. 2012, web, 26 Feb. 2016.
57 "USA and Canada – Aborted Fetal Cell Line Products and Ethical Alternatives," *Children of God for Life*, https://www.cogforlife.org/vaccineListOrigFormat.pdf, 2015, web, 01 Sept. 2015.
58 Tenpenny, Sherri, "The Truth About the Flu Shot," https://drtenpenny.com/the-truth-about-the-flu-shot/, NMA Media-Press, LLC., 2011, web, 12 April 2015.
59 Joel, Lord, Vaccine Resistance Movement, http://vaccineresistancemovement.org/?p=12642, January 2016, web, 08 Jan. 2016.
60 Humphries, Dr. Suzanne, "The Attack on Pregnant Mothers Escalates," http://www.vaccinationcouncil.org/2012/02/29/3013, 29 Feb. 2012, web, 02 May 2015.

without thimerosal.[61] It is ironic that pregnant women are warned not eat too much tuna; not to exercise too much; but to get a flu shot—and every other 'safe' medication that one needs. According to the National Vaccine Information Center in response to the warnings listed on the flu shot:

> The adult influenza vaccine injury claims are the leading claim submitted to the federal Vaccine Injury Compensation Program. [....] [T]here are no adequate and well-controlled studies in pregnant women and no animal data, which means that animal reproduction studies have not been conducted and it is not known whether these vaccines can cause fetal harm when administered to a pregnant woman or if they can affect pregnant mothers.

The response I was given by the pharmacist at Walgreens, where I received my flu shot when pregnant, might have been pulled directly from the U.S. government and posted online for those with concern to learn the "facts."[62] The "key facts" include indication that all should receive the flu vaccine, including babies of six months up and pregnant women. The flu shot is "the most important way of preventing seasonal influenza virus infections and potentially severe complications, including death." It is advised that children receive the nasal spray vaccine, though it has been proven to cause convulsions, narcolepsy, and neurological damage.[63] The insert of the vaccine indicates that immunosuppressed people should not have this version of the vaccine, nor should those with compromised immune systems be around others who have been given the flu vaccine.[64] I now wonder how many with the flu actually "caught" it from one who had been vaccinated with the nasal spray. It is a live, weakened version of the flu often given to children. The vaccine sheds in body fluids for a week (or more) after administration.[65]

Sadly, the issue of vaccination is unethical because the potential for harm and the ingredients are not addressed. Groups and individuals who speak against vaccines are said to be speaking against "truth" which is "science." I have been shocked when those I trust and admire for their intelligence dismiss valid research and claim the findings are not credible. I have found that it is easier for some who are quite smart to focus on what was mistaken in the way in which I say something regarding vaccination and its harm,

61 "Influenza Vaccine Package Inserts – Diseases and Vaccines – NVIC," *National Vaccine Information Center*, http://www.nvic.org/vaccines-and-diseases/Influenza/Influenza-Vaccine-Package-Inserts.aspx, 2015, web, 03 May 2015.
62 "Seasonal Influenza Vaccine Safety: A Summary for Clinicians," http://www.cdc.gov/flu/professionals/vaccination/vaccine_safety.htm, CDC, 7 Aug. 2015, web, 01 Sept. 2015.
63 "11 Year Old Boy Narcoleptic, Seizures, After Flu Vaccine," http://edgytruth.com/2015/09/07/11-year-old-boy-narcoleptic-seizures-after-flu-vaccine/, *The Edgy Truth*, 07 Sept. 2015, web, 08 Sept. 2015.
64 Mercola, Dr. Joseph, "43% of Americans Risked Their Brain Health for Flu Shots – Did You? A Flu Shot May Jeopardize Your Brain Health," http://articles.mercola.com/sites/articles/archive/2011/11/24/more-people-getting-flu-shots.aspx, 24 Nov. 2011, web, 03 Mar. 2015.
65 "Influenza Information – Diseases and Vaccines – NVIC," http://www.nvic.org/vaccines-and-diseases/influenza.aspx, NVIC, 2015, web, 31 Oct. 2015.

rather than listen to the greater truth concerning very real risk that smart medical people should look into and unravel through their scientific knowledge, as many others have.

It would benefit the world if we were willing to change our minds when the facts that what we have been taught do not align with what we see in our kids and experience in our own bodies. Mainstream media promotes articles from academia, government, and health care industries that argue in favor of vaccination, but why has the other side of the story not been investigated by the mainstream media? Who is lying?--and why? There is no gain in realizing harm in a common, in some cases mandatory, "health care" practice. There is much information floating around the Internet, but it is concerning that information written to explain other theories and counter-argue vaccination is not initially found on the Internet. Searches first pop up with a wealth of material from government and institution-supported sites, and the same "safe and effective" claim is recycled. It doesn't take much digging to find sources like *Natural News* and *Green Med.* that show another side of the story. Unfortunately, though the information is available, some dismiss it all together. "Vactruth lies," I have been told. In the course of my research these past few years, I haven't seen why those arguing against vaccines would bother, other than it is the truth and they wish to help the world. On the other hand, there is a lot to lose if one accepts the lies and accepts the need to unravel a faulty medical paradigm and change.

The website, *The History of Vaccines: An Educational Resource by the College of Physicians of Philadelphia*[66] is a perfect example of a source that shapes the story of vaccination according to our culture. For example, the page on "Ethical Issues and Vaccines" fails to mention vaccine ingredients, risks to the vaccinated, or the fact that diseases are higher in vaccinated populations. There is no mention of the many concerns raised about the link to autism and other conditions resulting from brain trauma / damage. It is stated that some may object to mandatory vaccination and place others at risk. No reasons are provided for this objection: "[I]n an effort to protect the greatest number of people, public health vaccine regulations may infringe upon individual autonomy and liberty."

Autonomy and liberty have little to do with the fact that I do not vaccinate because it is better for my body not to vaccinate as a result of lax safety standards and dangerous ingredients including animal and human cells, heavy metals, and peanut oil that can sensitize the body to peanuts and create allergy. The benefit of temporarily elevated antigens (which may not even indicate immunity, as the whole vaccine effectiveness is positioned upon) to some diseases in some people does not outweigh the potential risk of autism, brain damage, and death. There is no mention of the ethical objection that

---

66 "The History of Vaccines: An Educational Resource by the College of Physicians of Philadelphia," http://www.historyofvaccines.org/content/articles/ethical-issues-and-vaccines, The College of Physicians of Philadelphia, 2015, web, 05 June 2015.

others and I have to fetal stem cells injected into my body, or the bodies of my babies, or the risks of unavoidable trace amounts of foreign human DNA injected into another human being. Rather than legitimate ethical considerations, the argument segues to the ethical responsibility to vaccinate all equally. "From an ethical perspective, increasing the number of vaccine producers would greatly influence health positively. When vaccines are in short supply, medical providers must make decisions about who should be protected, and who must be left vulnerable to disease." This statement implies that vaccines protect, and individuals are all vulnerable to disease. It argues in typical blanket-form: as though *all* vaccines are safe and effective and *all* individuals are in need based on in-common vulnerability to disease. It fails to note that vaccines can actually cause diseases they are intended to provide immunity to, and that vaccines shed and spread disease among others. The problem that pervades health care with over-reliance on medications and a lack of attention to the individual is acute in the current program of vaccination.

There are exceptional medical doctors like Suzanne Humphries who resigned from her accomplished career to battle for the truth in regards to vaccination.[67] Health care has been hijacked by pharmaceutical companies and is making us sick, and some refuse to give in to the system, though it costs them much. Dr. Humphries was a sought-after nephrologist prior to 2009.[68] She left her success and a $300,000.00 income to become a "low-paid researcher, all because her integrity wouldn't allow her to turn a blind eye to what she was seeing in her practice." Truth doesn't change, how scientists see truth changes, she says. Unfortunately, medical professionals have a difficult time reconceptualizing immunity, which they have been trained to understand as related primarily to vaccination. Humphries says,

We have a highly profitable, lucrative religion that involves the government, industry, and academia. That religion is vaccination. People believe in vaccines. They will tell you, they believe in vaccines. But you ask them what they know about vaccines and it will be almost nothing. Medical schools are bereft of information on the history of vaccination, on the contents of them, and the potential problems. Doctors are really being systematically brainwashed. Not only that, but if doctors do start to see problems... wake up to it; do their own research, and buck the system, they risk being treated the way I was. I was well respected through the entire state of Maine. People were referring their patients to me. My colleagues would come to me with their medical problems... But once I started to argue against the practice of vaccination, I was automatically tossed into the category of a quack.

---

67 Humphries, Dr. Suzanne, *Dissolving Illusions: Disease, Vaccines, and the Forgotten History*, CreateSpace, 2013.
68 Roberts, Jeff, "The Forgotten History of Vaccines and Diseases Everyone Should Know," *Collective-Evolution*, January, 2015.

In an interview with Dr. Joseph Mercola, Humphries explains that she had been pro-vaccine. She vaccinated her patients, herself, and she believed what she had been taught in medical school. She worked with acutely ill patients. They suffered inflammatory diseases, and she did not want them to be vaccinated before she met with them. Her patients continued coming to her having been vaccinated right away when they were admitted for health care. She didn't understand why her order wasn't being observed and began to research medical literature on vaccines in such cases of immune suppressed patients. She found that there wasn't any literature on vaccines in patients who were acutely ill. She began to push harder that her patients not be vaccinated against her will until she met with them. As she began to research and change her mind on vaccination, she delved into the history of smallpox and polio.

Dr. Humphries was startled to realize that what she had been taught in medical school regarding these diseases was inaccurate. This history was complicated and people were ignorant of it. The smallpox vaccine developed before the human immune system was understood, and the vaccine actually came from a rumor that if a dairy maid were infected with a common cowpox virus, then she would not be susceptible to smallpox. Edward Jenner scrapped puss off the belly of a cow, sometimes goat genetic disease was also in there. Human pox was mixed in and some glycerin. It was the most unclean of all vaccines.[69] Many people developed smallpox from the vaccine, and the vaccine-derived smallpox virus was severe and many died. Statistics reveal that more people died that were vaccinated than those who died from the natural smallpox virus. The vaccine was stopped. In Leicester, England, the mayor and some health officials met in a town meeting and agreed that the vaccine would no longer be issued. At this point, because of sanitation and isolation, the smallpox disease was eliminated.

The history of polio has likewise been completely twisted, and understanding the history of polio and the polio vaccines shows us exactly why disease is not eradicated but worsened by vaccination. Neil Miller provides a critical assessment of the polio vaccine and details the history, efficacy, and long-term health-related consequences of integrating the polio vaccine into society.[70] Most in my grandparents' and parents' generations fear polio and believe that the polio vaccine prevents us from suffering the "iron lung" and horrific paralysis from poliomyelitis. Surprisingly, in the late 40s and into the 50s when polio was an epidemic in the U.S., vaccines, poor diet, and neurotoxins together provided a perfect climate for crippling effects of a disease that is actually benign in the absence of neurotoxic catalysts. As Miller, Humphries and others explain, injections increase one's susceptibility to poliomyelitis, and in the late 40s the pertussis and diphtheria vaccines were administered to the public. A diet of high sugar and starch also increases the harmful effects of the disease. In fact, polio was often thought to

---

69 Carrell, Dr. Jennifer Lee, *The Speckled Monster: A Historical Tale of Battling Smallpox*, Plume, 2004, explains that the original term "vaccine" was an inoculation against smallpox using a cowpox virus. "Vacca" means cow. The term has come to mean all inoculations against any disease.
70 Miller, Neil Z., "The Polio Vaccine: A Critical Assessment of its Arcane History, Efficacy, and Long-term Health-related Consequences," *Thinktwice Global Vaccine Institute*, Santa Fe, 2004, 239-251.

strike in the summer, precisely because of the high-sugar diet of ice cream, etc. that many enjoyed. Neurotoxic pesticides were also sprayed on people, food, and homes to keep disease-carrying mosquitos away.

Jim West writes about the history of polio and its correlation to the use of pesticides and other poisons.[71] The insecticide DDT (chlorophenoethane, dichloro-diphenyl-trichloroethane) was used to kill disease-carrying mosquitos in the 1950s. Other poisons such as Benzene hexachloride (BHC), lead, and arsenic, as well as DDT, cause paralysis, which has been diagnosed as "polio," according to West. There was a song with the jingle, "D-D-T is good for me," and the poison was spread on toast, sprayed all over children at the pool and playground, and used in American homes, and it was even found in human breast milk. At this time, Dr. Morton S. Biskind researched and reported that neurotoxins such as DDT could cause paralysis from central nervous system dysfunction caused by the chemical. Wayland J. Hayes and Edward R. Laws refuted Biskind's claims in their *Handbook of Pesticide Toxicology* (1991), calling Dr. Biskind a "heretic."

> Through this intellectually paralyzing atmosphere, Dr. Biskind had the composure to argue what he thought was the most obvious explanation for the polio epidemic: Central nervous system diseases (CNS) such as polio are actually the physiological and symptomatic manifestations of the ongoing government- and industry-sponsored inundation of the world's populace with central nervous system poisons. [....] When the population is exposed to a chemical agent known to produce in animals lesions in the spinal cord resembling those in human polio, and thereafter the latter disease increases sharply in incidence and maintains its epidemic character year after year, is it unreasonable to suspect an etiologic relationship?

Ten years later, Rachel Carson spoke out on the poison's destruction of environment and wildlife, but she did not extend her argument to humankind. There was too much controversy, too much resistance. But when nature is negatively affected, people are too.

Polio is a "passenger virus," and this means that the virus itself is oftentimes harmless. When there is an "accelerated genetic recombination", the biologic system is threatened. Pesticides and radiation can threaten the biological system of the virus and cause the manifestation of the disease. "It is ironic that common medical procedures such as chemotherapy, radiation therapy, and the use of toxic pharmaceuticals accelerate genetic recombination and thus the potential for a necessary virus proliferation." West writes:

---

71 West, Jim, "Pesticides and Polio: A Critique of Scientific Literature," http://www.westonaprice.org/health-topics/pesticides-and-polio-a-critique-of-scientific-literature/, *The Weston A. Price Foundation for Wise Traditions in Food, Farming, and the Healing Arts*, 8 Feb. 2003, web, 01 Sept. 2015.

[F]rom ancient times to the early 20th century, the symptoms and physiology of paralytic poliomyelitis were often described as the results of poisoning. It wasn't until the mid-19th century that the word 'poliomyelitis' became the designation for the paralytic effects of both severe poisoning and polio-like diseases assumed to be germ-caused. [....] Polio shows no movement independent from pesticide movement, as one would expect if it were caused by a virus. Both the medical and popular imaginations are haunted by the image of a virus that invades (or infects) and begins replicating to the point of producing disease. [....] The most obvious theory–pesticide causation–should be the dominant theory. But the opposite exists, a pervasive silence regarding pesticide causation juxtaposed against a steady stream of drama regarding virus causation. In light of the evidence presented herein, the silence could ultimately discredit mainstream medical science, institutions of the environmental movement, and the World Health Organization.

Miller explains the history of polio vaccine development, which helps one see why the vaccines themselves cause polio. The Salk vaccine used high amounts of formaldehyde, and other scientists and medical doctors advised against the vaccine because of the amount of formaldehyde, a known neurotoxin. The vaccine contained a live virus in 1954, which caused polio, and so Salk's vaccine for polio was reformulated with an attenuated, weakened or "dead" virus, in 1955. In 1958, the Sabin vaccine for polio was live and oral, and it was administered from 1958-2000. All cases of polio between 1960-2000 occurred from the Sabin live, oral polio vaccine, given with the belief that it would be more effective than Salk's vaccine (cases of polio were still occurring—from the vaccine, diets, and neurotoxins, some of which were in the vaccine itself). In the 1950s, there were more cases of polio than before the vaccination program, and this despite the change in the definition of "poliomyelitis" which was meant to narrow the disease diagnosis.

Vaccines for polio have always caused the disease, as Humphries explains. The injectable vaccine can theoretically provide blood immunity, if the virus is in the blood before it meets the central nervous system. The story of the development of the vaccine is quite telling, especially considering the recent news and the "threat" of two cases of polio in the Ukraine, for which health officials are encouraging international efforts to administer polio vaccines, which can ultimately cause polio viruses, as explained below. "Pharmaceutical companies are more than happy to help implement an 'outbreak response' in order to save the continent of Europe, all the while increasing the movement of their vaccine products. Private donors, Government funding, will race to respond by purchasing vaccines."[72]

---

72 "Polio Outbreak Declared in Europe," http://edgytruth.com/2015/09/04/polio-outbreak-declared-in-europe/, *The Edgy Truth*, 09 Sept. 2015, web, 10 Sept. 2015.

According to Humphries, to begin, a number of viruses cause paralysis, but prior to the vaccine, doctors diagnosed most instances of paralysis as "polio." In 1955, the live polio vaccine caused paralysis and injury of many, with three strains of the virus in the oral vaccine. Still, most people who had the vaccine recovered from symptoms of slight paralysis and fatigue (induced by the vaccine). According to Humphries, 95% of people who have the disease do not have symptoms. Of the five percent who do, only one percent become paralyzed. Ironically, everyone is to be vaccinated against polio in the U.S. Vaccination has led to polio outbreaks, and Humphries explains why this is so.

With the oral polio vaccination, a person hosts the virus and it can mutate or combine with other bowel viruses, creating new strains, often more virulent than others. The oral vaccine interrupted transmission of the wild form of polio, but propagated transmission of vaccine-derived virus. Though few healthy people given the vaccine develop polio, babies excrete the virulent poliovirus they had been injected with. This becomes a problem, especially for immunosuppressed people who may change a diaper or otherwise come in contact with the shedding poliovirus. Outbreaks of polio have occurred when people in other countries come to the States having been vaccinated with strains different from our vaccine. When people from other countries receive the oral vaccine and come to the States, they shed the highly virulent strain, and people here pass it around. Since the 1990s, our vaccine is injected, inactivated poliovirus, using one or two strains. This vaccine does not interrupt the propagation of the virus.

Statistics reveal that outbreaks occurred with global vaccination efforts (for example in 1955). Many think President Theodore Roosevelt had polio and campaigned to eradicate the disease, but the president did not likely have polio, according to Dr. Humphries. She argues that in fact his campaigns correlated with increased rates of the polio disease in places where the vaccine was administered. In another example, Bill Gates polio vaccine program in India caused 47,500 deaths.[73] There continues much propaganda that suggests a healthier society because of the widespread use of vaccines. For example, just consider the recent (February 2016) photograph posted in Catholic News Service of Pope Francis of the Catholic Church administering an oral polio vaccine, which includes aborted fetal stem cells, to a small boy. For the specific reasons, which follow, this is clearly inaccurate.

Dr. Humphries specializes in infant epigenetics. She claims that vaccinating babies tinkers with an infant's immune system and plants "cluster bombs" that may later explode. She says that research now shows that we are not victims to our genes. Each person has a unique response to each vaccine, which is why there is no compensation possible for vaccine harm. In many, we won't know the harm immediately. Many argue vaccines do not cause autism, cancer, developmental delays, and many other ills, but we

---

73   Adl-Tabatabai, Sean, "Bill Gates: Polio Vaccine Program Causes 47,500 Deaths," http://yournewswire.com/bill-gates-polio-vaccine-program-causes-47500-deaths/, *Your News Wire*, 09 Feb. 2015, web, 01 Mar. 2015.

see that they do. Humphries claims:

> Most doctors are uninformed and therefore cannot give informed consent.
>
> [Vaccines] can have tumorigenic kidney cells of a cocker spaniel in it. It can have human fetal cells with retroviruses. [It can have] aluminum, which is one of the most horrible things to inject into any sort of life form, especially into a muscle... Parents really need to know that their doctors are not informed and therefore they cannot give informed consent, and that they really need to think about it because you cannot unvaccinate. The fear of, 'Oh, what if my child gets a disease'—that's where knowing the history is really important because what we're talking about is under which conditions people become susceptible. That's really more important than transmission. Because, yes, measles transmits very rapidly through the population, but it actually has a lot of benefits to the immune system—so much so that they're using it to treat cancer today.

As Dr. Humphries explains, the history of vaccines for smallpox and polio, when studied in the contexts of the diseases themselves, undoes the entire argument in favor of vaccination. Vaccines have not lowered disease rates; they have increased diseases and worsened them. People want the truth, and we want to realize the truth concerning vaccination before vaccines are mandated. Time is of the essence, but it takes quite a while for minds to truly change. I pray that there is enough time to understand the grave implications of vaccination before more states enforce mandates.

In society at large, health care workers are educated to believe in vaccines as a public safety measure. They are led to surmise that only those who are ignorant would deny the benefits of "immunization." A young nurse mentioned to my sister that they have meetings where health care workers discuss the growing unrest concerning vaccination. She and her colleagues are encouraged to perceive parents with informed reasons for exempting their children from vaccines as negligent and erroneous. Workers are discouraged from understanding many people's growing resolve not to vaccinate. Perhaps some do anyways, despite being told that vaccines are safe and effective. Perhaps some do anyways because they have seen harm occur after vaccination. Many times, patients do not react immediately after vaccination, and with the silencing of scientists and doctors who have given voice to the various ills caused by vaccination, health care providers may think that there is no evidence to suggest vaccine harm.

When we begin to learn of the gobs of money made by pharmaceutical companies and the U.S. government, it is not only infuriating; it is a horrific assault on the sanctity of life. Blind trust in health care is obliterated, though this does not necessary impact negatively my appreciation for health care providers. It is important to realize that health care workers have been misinformed, and the theory of vaccination as safe and effective is supported with skewed evidence and scientific theories that are false. I sincerely believe that doctors, nurses, aides and others are working diligently to help people; unfortunately, they are doing so according to the rubrics of their training. I will never forget when I asked my son's allergist if vaccines might cause these allergies that kids are "getting." He stopped to think, and his response was open: "I gave your son the flu shot." He had a look on his face that did not throw out my claim, or accept it. His initial response was one of responsibility to my son's wellbeing. This same allergist gave me his home phone number and spoke with me for over an hour one evening when our son had a life-threatening reaction to sugar-snap peas.

Our culture is being fed a lie in the name of health care, and in no way should a Christian abide it. From a spiritual perspective, what profits the body, profits the soul and injecting even trace amounts of aborted fetal stem cells harms our lives. The specific ingredients of each vaccine, including fetal stem cells, may seem like a necessary evil, when a person is unaware of the ineffectiveness of the vaccine to protect against disease and the potential for harm associated with vaccination. I read an article written by an Orthodox priest who argued that even if vaccines included aborted stem cells, just like war, there were times when one chose the lesser of the evils.[74] His argument justified vaccines under the faulty conclusion that they keep children healthy. My research into vaccines, and many others' who have studied the science of vaccine production and the culture surrounding the implementation of the vaccination program in the U.S. (and elsewhere) since the inception of vaccines in the 1900s, shows that vaccination carries substantial risks and there is really only one benefit: to feed pharmaceutical companies' cash cow.

For mothers and fathers, it may not be difficult to believe the science that proves vaccines ineffective and harmful (when it is shared with us), if we pay attention to the state of children's health in our developed nation. It is little wonder why this is so when we learn of the specific harmful ingredients, which can be read from the insert of the vaccine. Doctors do not present this insert to patients, though patients may ask, but we have access to the information at http://vactruth.com/vaccine-inserts/.

Infants are vaccinated without discussion of potential side effects. Sometimes nurses enter the exam room with a tray of vaccines and there isn't so much as an announcement of which shots are being administered. It is assumed that the doctor has ordered what the infant needs. It is believed that the vaccine program will keep kids well. Parents trust their doctors. That is, until something happens that causes a parent to reconsider the normal way of vaccinating children. I understand this blind trust. My boys were vaccinated, and at the time, I had thought that it was in their best interest. I hadn't had any information, or experience, to suggest otherwise.

---

74 Obregon, Fr. Ernesto, "Vaccination, Fetal Cell Cultures, and Orthodoxy," http://myocn.net/should-orthodox-parents-vaccinate-children/, *The Sounding, Orthodox Christian Network*, 23 June 2014, web, 07 June 2015.

The mom who goes to her family pediatrician is not informed, as she ought to be even though medical investigators as well as health care providers have spoken out[75] against vaccination since inception of programs to vaccinate mass populations in the 1900s. The news a mother views when she returns from the pediatrician confirms her choice to get the shots at all costs, as horrific reports of "life-threatening" diseases such as the measles plague her thoughts. Never mind that her mother had it, along with all of her siblings and friends on the street, and lived through the week without much care. Many more today are dealing with illnesses and allergies than the few who didn't bounce back from the measles.

When I met with a physician and advocate of holistic medicine and she said that the healthiest kids she sees are not vaccinated, I balked. My boys had been vaccinated. They were pretty healthy. How dare she. After watching my two girls develop (three and five) without having been vaccinated, I understand the doctor's comment. There is resilience to my girls, and even when they become ill (which is rare), they mend quickly, without complications of infection, bronchitis, or even bowel troubles. As kids, they'll be ill, but in my experience, they are healthier than my vaccinated boys were at their ages. They also develop "normal" speech and motor skills. They are able to pay attention, to speak, and show interest in books and stories. My three-year-old recites prayers. Her memory is strong. Of course, listening to her sing the alphabet and mix together her version of stories, prayers, and yelling at her brother (a sing-song after nap), it's hard to say what all is happening in her brain. The point is, kids should be able to eat foods and speak, they should be able to run and laugh without the ailments of stomach conditions and too-frequent illnesses. Vaccines cannot make children healthy, and they may even cause future problems, such as cancer[76] and infertility.[77, 78] The inserts of most vaccines state that it "has not been evaluated for its carcinogenic or mutagenic potentials or impairment of fertility." It seems we should be told about these risks before vaccinating our children, but we are not.

A friend and young woman studying to become a doctor sent me an instant message with an article attached on microbiology to "inject science into my understanding of vaccination." As the argument goes, those who oppose vaccination, oppose "science." In reality, many scientists speak against the misleading science in support of vaccines.[79] Dr.

75 Jordan, Patrick, "Allergy-Immunity-Hypersensitivity and Vaccines: The Hidden Link," http://vactruth.com/2012/09/05/allergy-and-vaccines/, Vactruth, 5 Sept. 2012, web, 01 April 2015.
76 Aufderheide, Jeffry John, "3 Filthy Truths About Vaccines and Cancer," http://thelibertybeacon.com/2013/09/05/13-filthy-truths-about-vaccines-and-cancer-1846/, Liberty Beacon, 05 Sept. 2013, web, 08 Sept. 2015.
77 England, Christina, "Vaccines Can Cause Infertility," http://vactruth.com/2013/07/20/vaccines-can-cause-infertility/, Vactruth, 20 July 2013, web, 08 Sept. 2015.
78 Hawkes, Dr. Dave, "A scientist answers all your questions about the HPV vaccination," http://www.mamamia.com.au/news/hpv-vaccination/, Mamamia Women's Network, 22 Dec. 2013, web, 13 July 2015.
79 "Dr. Andrew Wakefield Calls Out CDC on 'Vaccine Science,'" http://edgytruth.com/2015/08/19/dr-andrew-wakefield-calls-out-cdc-on-vaccine-science/#, Edgy Truth, 04 Aug. 2015, web, 10 Aug. 2015.

Gary Null and Richard Gale go so far as to argue that the vaccine paradigm is deliberately flawed. In their article, they use science to back their riveting claims.[80]

In Dr. Null's and Mr. Gale's article, they present statistics to argue that vaccines are deliberately flawed, and the facts they present speak loud and clear to show the following:

1. Largest outbreaks of infectious diseases are within the most highly vaccinated populations.
2. Influenza vaccine is ineffective in preventing flu.
3. Influenza vaccine causes harm to the elderly but it is continually marketed to them.
4. The mumps vaccine is useless and causes harm in adults.
5. A fully vaccinated woman through secondary transmission initiated the Disneyland measles outbreak.
6. There is more whooping cough among those vaccinated with the pertussis vaccine.
7. The rubella vaccine causes depression.
8. Hepatitis B vaccine causes multiple sclerosis.
9. Rotavirus vaccine (2010) may have been contaminated with a baboon endogenous virus.
10. The human papilloma vaccine is fraudulent, and cervical cancer may not even be (other sources confirm it is not) caused by HPV (it also leads to "higher oncogene expression" and "the vaccine is driving the evolution of viral virulence" similar to what is observed in pertussis, mumps and measles).
11. Chickenpox vaccine increases disease rates.

In conclusion, of their excellent and concise article, they state,

> The vaccine establishment is desperate. The ghosts of their fraudulent science manipulated research, misleading propaganda across mainstream media and in the blogosphere are returning to haunt them. The pro-vaccine pundits are rapidly losing credibility as increasing numbers of parents and young adults educate themselves about vaccine efficacy and their health risks. If it were left for an open scientific debate between pro-vaccinators and those opposing vaccines, the former would not have sound science on their side. It is time for a national debate to end vaccine madness. As further research emerges, as the vaccine paradigm is further stripped away, future generations will be looking back upon vaccination as a barbaric, primitive practice.

---

80   Null, Dr. Gary, Richard Gale, "Vaccine McCarthyism. What if the Vaccine Paradigm itself is Deliberately Flawed?," http://www.globalresearch.ca/vaccine-mccarthyism-what-if-the-vaccine-paradigm-itself-is-deliberately-flawed/5427768, Global Research, 28 Jan. 2015, web, 01 Sept. 2015.

Currently, more and more experts such as doctors and scientists are speaking out against the atrocities of the current vaccination program in the U.S. Additionally, whistleblowers, or those who worked within "Big Pharma," are testifying to the fact that pharmaceutical companies fund and support institutions of higher learning, healthcare, and the government (such as funding politicians who support mandatory vaccinations). Paying attention to this news, which is not broadcast by mainstream media, I have had many, many concerns and questions. How could this happen and how could so many not be aware of it happening?

Current media aims to silence whistleblowers like Brandy Vaughan, a former sales rep for the vaccine maker Merck & Co.[81] However, she, among others, realizes that mandatory vaccination represents sinister control and harms society. Their consciences won't let them remain silent, though it may cost reputation, career, and even personal safety.

Vaughan details how vaccine companies use vaccines for massive profit. She says that "mandatory vaccination is for profit and not public health." After researching the safety of vaccines, she found that they contain known toxins that can cause neurological damage, such as aluminum. She also tells how vaccine makers do not create the same safety studies for vaccines as they do for other drugs. "This lack of true safety research of vaccines combined with the known adverse reactions to vaccinations has helped Brandy decide never to vaccinate her own child. Brandy says giving children a vaccine is like playing Russian roulette with our children and that mandatory vaccination is simply a way for vaccine makers to profit off our children."

After researching vaccines in the U.S. compared with other developed countries, she found that children in the U.S. are given twice as many vaccines than most other countries, and children here have the highest incidence of SIDS, asthma, food allergies, ADHD, childhood leukemia, and diabetes type one. The true health crisis, as she notes, is that kids are sicker here than in other developed countries, and this is so despite spending more per capita on health care. This information led her to believe that vaccines are not for public health but for pharmaceutical company profit.

The thing about vaccines is that you don't have to do the same rigorous safety studies as you do for other pharmaceutical drugs because they're classified as a public health measure vs. a pharma drug. For vaccines, they have a totally different type of safety study. It's very short in duration. It's not double blind placebo-based. [....] [I]t's very easy to manipulate the data and present that as something that's safe. If you really look into the studies and look into the toxicity of the adjuvants and the additives, you realize that the safety studies

---

81   Cook, Larry, "Former Merck Rep Says Mandatory Vaccination Is For Profit and Not Public Health – YouTube," https://m.youtube.com/watch?v=LUdiwgHMQs, Stop Mandatory Vaccination, 05 Aug. 2015, web, 06 Aug. 2015.

are not proving safety at all. In fact, there are many studies on the other side showing that a lot of the additives in vaccines are very toxic, especially to children who have very immature immune systems.

The question Brandy faced was the same predominant question I had: Why is this happening? She explains that pharmaceutical companies have recently lost their patent on "blockbuster drugs" in the past few years, and they aim to profit from vaccines. There are mandatory vaccine bills in 138 states (throughout the world) to ensure that this happens. Vaccines are easier to get on the market with less rigorous safety studies and pharmaceutical companies do not have any liability for vaccines. For these reasons, pharmaceutical companies consider vaccines the drug of choice for the market.

Why do we not hear about this if it is true? She explains that the U.S. is one of only two countries in the world that allows pharmaceutical companies to advertise directly to consumers. The pharmaceutical companies provide the media with 30-40 % of their advertising dollars, and so they are able to control what is said, and what is silenced. Vaughn explains that many journalists and stories have been censored. In fact, many initial CDC scientists were imported from Germany and had been Nazi doctors and scientists in WWII, according to S.D. Wells, cited below. Some of these individuals had been close allies to Adolf Hitler and were responsible for human experimentation, murder, and slavery.[82] Knowing this fact shakes my trust in the CDC. Vaughn argues a CDC whistleblower was silenced when he came out in 2014 saying the CDC covered up data showing that the MMR vaccine does in fact cause neurological damage (autism).[83] She goes on to tell of stories in other countries where vaccine makers have been sued for injury and death, prompting other countries to pull off their markets certain vaccines: Gardasil in Japan and Spain, Prevnar in China, and rotavirus in France.

The media is a very powerful source of information and influences society in profound ways. Nonetheless, vaccine harm can seem even obvious, once one connects the dots between the kids that have been vaccinated and their frequent colds and flus and those who have not and their infrequent bouts with illnesses. I have wondered how doctors and others in health care have not been more aware of the harm of vaccines. Vaughn responds:

Pharmaceutical companies spend 18 billion annually marketing directly to consumers through mainstream media. Yet they spend six times that marketing to doctors through health insurance plans, through educational conferences, through materials, through studies that are published in medical journals, all

---

82 "The CDC and CIA: A Close and Sick Relationship | 2012: What's the 'real' truth?" https://jhaines6.wordpress.com/2014/08/28/cdc-and-cia-a-close-and-sick-relationship/, Wordpress Blog, 28 Aug. 2014, web, 07 June 2015.
83 "CDC Whistleblower: CDC Covered Up MMR Vaccine Link to Autism in African American Boys," http://healthimpactnews.com/2014/cdc-whistleblower-cdc-covered-up-mmr-vaccine-link-to-autism-in-african-american-boys/, Health Impact News, 18 Aug. 2014, web, 08 Oct. 2015.

these types of things. [....]

Today's American government seems not to protect us from the obvious ills of pharmaceutical companies that desire profit over public health. This may be a result of our current government serving as a sort of corporation[84]—bought by powerful shareholders whose greed for money harms us. Vaughn argues:

> We have a very broken system. Our vaccine system in the U.S. is broken. We cannot mandate something when there are so many unanswered questions and so many things that are going on behind the scenes that people aren't aware of. [...] [In vaccines] there is aluminum, formaldehyde, fetal cells, animal cells. There are a lot of things in there that other countries A, ban from being ingested and therefore have vaccines that don't include these ingredients, and B, have unknown consequences that we have no data on right now.

Shortly after Brandy Vaughn aired the YouTube that included the above information, she had break-ins to her home and various threats to her safety. I was deeply distraught over the truth that was beginning to convict me that vaccines were for profit and not public health, and the reality of the extreme power of Big Pharma. I was amazed by the many who seemed outraged against changing their minds concerning vaccination, even after hearing incriminating information, such as Vaughn's researched claims and personal experiences. It seemed that until a person or their loved one was harmed, they would continue following the vaccination program set in motion by pharmaceutical companies. I also worried about this woman who was brave enough to speak out. My friend Stephen Muse emailed me in response to my fear. He commented that "corporate thugs" with power and money act above the law and manipulate the law. They care less about getting caught for say, killing a whistleblower, than they care for making money. In these cases, corporations act like a sociopath interested in profit. He writes,

> Mammon has no conscience. Only people who run corporations can change things if they have a conscience. But the 'system' whose prime directive is to make profits for stakeholders, will always push against that kind of morality with its own version. Research in 70 different countries shows that those who chase after money become less philanthropic, more manipulative, less empathic and more destructive of the environment.

Learning what I have about vaccination history, ingredients, and profit has led me to distrust the health care as a "system." It is painful to realize that those who should know often don't, and it can be frustrating when others fail to consider the risks involved in vaccination—and it is especially gut-wrenching when others seem not to care. There are

---

84 "Governments Have Descended to the Level of Mere Private Corporations," http://anticorruptionsociety.files.wordpress.com/2014/05/clearfield-doctrine.pdf, Clearfield Doctrine, May 2014, web, 01 Sept. 2015.

endless reasons we must care. It isn't only our health and our children's, it is society's, and the world's. In her fresh realization of the harm of the current vaccination program in the U.S., my sister shared very strong and persuasive arguments with dentists and others where she works as a dental hygienist, friends, and family. "Can't we all read?" she asked me in astonishment. It takes time, I mentioned. And people don't want to believe, I added. She said that it is like telling people about God who refuse to listen and believe.

Some wonder what the big deal is concerning the vaccine debate because our culture has been led to believe that vaccines protect us from disease: end of story. I had a conversation with a friend and a PhD in the sciences who mentioned to me that all vaccines aim to do is stimulate a process of immunity without having to make people seriously ill. This is a good thing, as the argument goes.

"Why would one rather build natural immunity than vaccinate?"

"Because it is better to make one nutritionally sufficient than to vaccinate, especially considering the ways that vaccines are currently manufactured with aborted fetal stem cells and adjuvants that can sensitize one to allergies, cause brain damage, and even death."

"What if we faced a communicable disease epidemic?"

"In short, I am more fearful of current vaccines than the diseases themselves because of the ingredients and current lax testing regulations, and because of the absolute bias in media, which counters my personal experiences." If only the conversation began and ended so smoothly. In truth, I was in tears, my friend was irritated, and there was a lot of nonsense muddling up the main points we each had. It is difficult for a mother, even one with a PhD in argument, to make sense when talking with a scientist (also a caring father and Christian) who believes the current vaccine paradigm. I hadn't then known the history of the smallpox and polio vaccines and the statistics of disease outbreaks that correlate with administration of vaccinations in particularly telling ways. Knowing that smallpox disappeared because of isolation of those infected and improved sanitation, without the use of the vaccine, and that polio paralysis occurs in only one percent of five percent of entire populations exposed to the virus, I am certain that it is better to risk disease than vaccination.

My scientist friend asked if I understood "germ theory," which I had not. His question prompted my investigation into differences between infection theories. In "Infection Theories Contrasted, Germs vs. Toxins[85]," a simple break down of the argument is:

---

85 "Germs Theory vs. Toxins Theory," http:healingtools.tripod.com/gvt.html, Total Health Associates, 01 April 2015, web, 04 June 2015.

GERMS – Louis Pasteur	TOXINS – Antoine Bechamp
Disease arises from Micro-Organisms, originating OUTSIDE of the Body.	The susceptibility to Disease arises from conditions WITHIN the Cells of the Body.
Micro-Organisms should be GUARDED AGAINST and DESTROYED to PREVENT Disease.	Micro-Organisms are BENEFICIAL and LIFE-SUSTAINING, if the Body is kept CLEAN from Toxins.
The appearance and function of specific Micro-Organisms is CONSTANT.	The appearance and function of Micro-Organisms CHANGES, when the Host Organism is injured, either mechanically, biochemically or emotionally.
EVERY Disease is associated with a particular Micro-Organism.	EVERY Disease is associated with a particular Condition.
Micro-Organisms are PRIMARY causal agents.	Micro-Organisms ONLY become associated with Disease, when the Cells become TOXIFIED.
Disease is INEVITABLE and can STRIKE ANYBODY.	Disease arises from Conditions of increased TOXICITY.
To PREVENT and CURE Diseases, it is NECESSARY to build defenses and to DESTROY Pathogenic Micro-Organisms.	PREVENTING or CURING consists of cleaning TOXICITY from the Body in a way that does NO HARM.

I believe the toxin theory of disease explains most accurately my first son's peanut allergy, acquired through vaccination during an inopportune time in his development. Most in the West have been trained to accept the germ theory and believe that vaccines prevent diseases by destroying "pathogenic micro-organisms." Those whose studies support toxin theory, and there are an increasing number of medical doctors and scientists whose research shows why vaccination is not helpful to the body, are essentially defamed and pushed out of the mainstream "system." Two prime illustrations are Dr. Sherri Tenpenny and Dr. Andrew Wakefield, both of whom have had tremendous success healing patients and helping them obtain fuller degrees of wellness.

The government protects vaccine manufacturers. Currently, the manufacturers of vaccines and the government report problems, injuries, and deaths associated with vaccinations.[86] Laws are in place to protect vaccine companies, and even if vaccines are attributed as a cause of harm, vaccine companies are protected from lawsuits. In 1986, the government to settle claims of vaccine injury established the National Vaccine Injury Compensation Program (referred to as the vaccine court). Tim Gihring reports[87] that in 1990, three quarters of the claims were related to the DTP vaccine (diphtheria, tetanus, and pertussis). The government provided multimillion-dollar settlements to families of those injured. Some of these children had severe brain damage caused by encephalitis after vaccination. In 2011, the British Medical Journal declared a study of vaccines and autism, headed by researcher Andrew Wakefield, fraudulent. The conclusion was that there are occasional side effects from vaccines, but not autism. In the same year, "the U.S. Supreme Court shielded drug companies from all liability for harm caused by vaccines mandated by government when companies could have made a safer vaccine." The companies who sell vaccines in America: Merck, Wyeth, Lederle, Connaught "blackmailed Congress" by threatening to stop the sale of vaccines in America, "unless a law was passed giving them complete immunity from prosecution."[88] By placing such limitations on patients' rights following vaccination, companies producing vaccines do not develop safer, better products. Naturopathic doctor, Jared Zeff, disapproves of the current vaccination program because of the harm that it may cause children and the lack of research on this harm.[89] With the threat of mandating vaccines, this is a genuine concern for each of us.

Unfortunately, esteemed medical professionals who work to communicate the harm of vaccination by explaining the ways that injecting vaccines and adjuvants cause harm to individuals and to the society at large, must also speak against the United States government's affiliated organizations such as the CDC. As a result, many whistleblowers are defamed, called quacks, and falsely accused of profiting by misleading individuals. There seems an agenda to rid society of those who dissent from the current goals of health care. Currently, nine holistic doctors in good health have unexpectedly gone missing, later to be found dead[90], cautioning others from speaking to the public.[91] "The

---

86   Wells, S.D. "Health Basics: The 11 Most Toxic Vaccine Ingredients and their Side Effects," http://m.naturalnews.com/news/035431_vaccine_ingredients_side_effects_MSG.html, Natural News, 29 February 2012, web, 04 June 2015.
87   Gihring, Tim, "The Refusers: Getting your shots used to be as American as motherhood and apple pie. Now a small but vocal group is saying no—with deadly consequences," http://www.minnesotamonthly.com/January-2012/The-Refusers/, Minnesota Monthly, January 2012, web, 04 April 2015.
88   Fisher, Barabara, "No Pharma Liability? No Vaccine Mandates—NVIC Newsletter," http://www.nvic.org/NVIC-Vaccine-News/March-2011/No-Pharma-Liability—No-Vaccine-Mandates-.aspx,National Vaccine Information Center, March 2011, web, 01 Sept. 2015.
89   Salmon Creek Clinic | Naturopathic Healthcare, http://salmoncreekclinic.com/, 2015, web, 15 May 2015.
90   Elizabeth, Erin, "Shocking Update: Another holistic doctor found dead in Florida bringing the total to 9," http://theheartysoul.com/shocking-update-another-holistic-doctor-found-dead-in-florida-bringing-the-total-to-9/, The Hearty Soul, 25 July 2015, web, 26 July 2015.
91   Bolen, Tim, "Is Big Pharma Murdering Our Cutting-Edge Doctors? Yes, Of Course They Are... Why? They've Tried Everything Else to Control the Dialogue,"

Father of Medical Freedom," Dr. Robert Rowen[92], among others, argues that the dark truth is found by following the money-trail. Most parents aren't interested in doing this when they visit their pediatrician for a well check with their new baby.

Changing my mind on vaccines was a process that occurred over a few years. At first, I blatantly did not think that vaccination was a serious risk for the healthy majority of people. Ultimately, before I realized the harm of vaccination, I thought the benefits out-weighed the risks, and I trusted doctors. Initially, when my husband brought home a video of a mother whose daughter died from encephalitis after her vaccinations at two-months, I wasn't all that moved. It seemed a freak incident, and I was sorry for this family, but it couldn't happen to many—because if there were real harm, then vaccines would not be routinely given to children. I believed the "vaccine paradigm" set in place by the pharmaceutical companies—who fund the media and institutions of higher learning and health care. I hadn't a reason not to because I wasn't aware of the many reasons my husband began to introduce. At the time, distrusting all of "Them" seemed on the brink of lunacy to me. I was certainly not a conspiracy theorist, even though my husband has a paper hanging on a bulletin board in the basement stating a conspiracy theorist is a derogatory term used to describe a critical thinker. The statement was prideful, arrogant. Like "They" were more informed than "Them." I didn't feel the need to engage a battle of ideas that seemed removed and insignificant. I was wrong.

Unless people learn about the harm of vaccinations and the control that the pharmaceutical companies have on health care, the current vaccination program will continue to harm us with the anticipated push of over 300 more vaccines in the making and plans to mandate them.[93] If we do not make a stand now, by objecting to doctors who want to vaccinate us and our children, by writing to our senators in protection of our civil liberties and freedom of medical choice, than we will be absorbed into a policed state that mandates what we do with our bodies.

As mentioned, I discredited my husband for a couple of years as he began to doubt the efficacy and safety of the current vaccination program. I wanted to speak with an expert and get the facts, and it was when he led us to one that I began to delve into this topic with an open mind. Three years ago, my husband and I met with Dr. Sherri Tenpenny, a medical doctor and specialist in muscular and skeletal systems and an outstanding holistic medicine practitioner in Ohio. She is a remarkable physician and highly credentialed, and her views are strong and founded. Some find her militant, but it is for good reason that she speaks with such confidence. She has studied medicine, worked with many young people and their families, and followed closely the worldwide

---

http://www.bolenreport.com/autism/antivaccine%20yes13.htm, Bolen Report, 26 Sept. 2015, web, 29 Sept. 2015.

92 Http://www.docrowen.com/, Home, web, 10 Aug. 2015.
93 Tenpenny, Dr. Sherri, "Healthy People 2020 And the Decade of Vaccines," www.drtenpenny.com/2015/03/09/healthy-people-2020-and-the-decade-of-vaccines/#, 09 Mar. 2015, web, 01 July 2015.

vaccination program. Her knowledge and concern emboldens her, and she is strong as steal. She argues that the government has had a plan to increase vaccinations and limit its citizens' freedom for 35 years.[94] She explains that the measles hysteria in all 50 states corresponded with the introduction of the mandatory vaccine bills to restrict and or remove vaccine exemptions (religious or philosophical). She argues "Healthy People" is a plan for controlling the health of citizens in all 50 states and began 35 years ago. In 2010, collaborates from all over the world came together with a global commitment to immunize, calling 2020 the decade of vaccines. There are currently "300 vaccines in the developmental pipeline," according to Tenpenny. She quotes from the 2010 meeting and states the dire effect:

> 'The National Vaccine Plan, developed by the U.S. Department of Human Services (HSS), is the roadmap for a 21st century vaccine and immunization enterprise.' It lays bare the incestuous public-private relationship between the pharmaceutical and vaccine manufacturers, the U.S. government, and the World Health Commission.

The plan includes government funding, supply and distribution of vaccines and pro-vaccine information pieces. All health care workers will be vaccinated. Requiring health care workers (and volunteers) to be vaccinated is a way to ensure those tending our wellness are on board with vaccination—or they are ill or dead as a result of having been vaccinated. Even if they are vaccine-injured, many will believe other causes for their illnesses. In every case, those who work in the field are pigeonholed into sharing the government's pro-vaccination position. If a person's career depends on being fully vaccinated, it becomes even trickier to question the status-quo and realize the serious problems with an intentionally flawed vaccine paradigm. Still, when problems obviously relate to vaccination, such individuals speak out, as has been seen in recent news (often delivered via non-mainstream venues). The goal seems to be a united pro-vaccine health care system, but many are now aware of problems caused by the vaccine agenda. There is resistance, despite the ridicule.

My children and I are the first generations that will have lived and learned the ill effects of vaccinating for HPV (human papillomavirus), shingles and rotavirus, the flu, and meningitis B, among other additional vaccines that are in the works. In our culture of vaccination, more are being pushed, and the harm is alarming. Many educated parents do not even realize that more vaccines are on the market and administered to children today than even a generation ago in my childhood. A simple chart of vaccine history[95] shows the radical increase in vaccines: in the 1940s, DTP and smallpox were given, and some children had four shots before two years of age. By the 1980s, eight shots were given before a child was two, and there were never more than two shots

---

94 "Healthy People 2020 And the Decade of Vaccines."
95 "Vaccination Myths: Contradictions between Medical Science and Immunization Policy," Natural News, Sprout Social Photos, 2015, web, 01 Oct. 2015.

administered at a time. It's shocking to see that by 2012, 14 shots, with 49 doses, were given to children by the age of six. Today, even more vaccines are advised up through pre-teen years, as one can view on the CDC list of recommended "immunizations," with boosters even as an adult. In fact, in 2013, vaccines for shingles, rotavirus, and child flu and in 2015, meningitis B were added. Today, children are given 49 doses of 14 different vaccines by the age of six, and they are given 70 doses of 16 vaccines by the age of 18. Additionally, more vaccines are on the horizon with an aggressive agenda to sell them to all in America.

I believe doctors help patients and are good intentioned. The best of them continue to investigate ways to increase wellness, and such good doctors are willing to change their minds when experience and research do not match up. Many doctors are not informed on vaccination, and parents must be vigilant for the sake of their children. When my husband and I met with Dr. Tenpenny, I had full intentions to vaccinate my baby. After talking with her for a good two hours, I agreed to continue researching before vaccination. Towards the end of our conversation, the doctor mentioned to my husband, "We have a convert." Thinking back on it, the conversion metaphor is appropriate. Changing one's mind on vaccination is a kind of conversion—it is a changed perspective, and it requires faith. My conviction has developed as I have read and listened to many experts who are speaking out against vaccinations. I have also become more certain that the current vaccine program is intentionally flawed by life experiences: speaking with pediatricians, other parents, friends, and family, and listening to the painfully biased mainstream news.

The tone of the vaccine debate persuades my conversion, as well, just as it had when I was converting to Orthodox Christianity. Those who speak up against vaccines are generally humble. In part, this is so because accepting the painful horrors of an established practice in health care that harms the most innocent among us, babies and infants, as well as those who are already in weakened condition, tends to press down upon a person's sense of confidence in the goodness at work in this world. Many may learn about vaccine risks, but those who accept that wellness is not coming through the vaccine, as we have been and are still told; realize this with attention to their own and others' bodies and spirits. Those who perceive loss are not arrogant but humbled. Those who are silencing voices that tell them what to think and aiming to realize what is honestly at stake are humbled. Especially when Christians who are scientists, such as Dr. Jay Wile claims that he is, assert that vaccines do not contain fetal tissue (though in his argument he admits there is a "grain of truth" in the claim that vaccines do contain fetal stem cells from two aborted babies back in the 1960s).[96] With a calloused heart, it may seem that there is difference between cells and tissue from an abortion, but the moral dilemma remains consistent in both cases: life is taken and used for a medication that

---

96 Wile, Dr. Jay, "Vaccines DO NOT Contain Fetal Tissue,"
http://locus.umdnj.edu/nia/nia_cgi/display.cgi?AG05965, *Proslogion: Thoughts from a scientist who is a Christian (not a Christian Scientist)*, 2009, web, 07 Oct. 2015.

can harm. Unfortunately, the fact is that aborted babies are being used in over 21 vaccines.

I am tempted to be angry and express outrage over this issue, but this fails to convey the greater message at hand. God is the Giver of Life, and retribution is His. Many simply do not know that there is potential harm and that there are fetal cells used in vaccinations. Many do not realize that many social issues are directly related to our health care practices of vaccination. Some have wondered who I am to say that I do know, and that the message I have is the right one. Certainly, people have been convicted of truths that are not true before.

I do not claim infallibility. I am a sinner trying to understand the Truth, against which there are many distractions and temptations. I have my experiences to offer, which include seeking out information and reflecting on situations with children all around me, including my own. I seek discernment in my body and spirit in genuine prayer with the Giver of Life. I aim for humility and wisdom, which in faith I acknowledge as only possible in a personal relationship with Jesus Christ. I do not seek Science. I seek God. This means that Life and its Giver are more valuable to me than any lesson, theory, or earthly teaching. Often Truth fails to make sense to me at a given time, but with faith and through life experiences, God allows understanding on the level of the whole body. Through the mind, heart, and soul, a person can understand things in powerful ways. Each will be held accountable for what she heard, believed, and chose to do. When we know better, we must do better—and doing better in this life is intricately tied to preserving the sanctity of life in small and great ways.

When I converted to holy Orthodoxy, I did so because I felt the presence of love in those who practiced the Faith. I converted because I experienced and came to appreciate that good could increase in the world: in others, in myself, in the universe, and that I could contribute to this growth as an Orthodox Christian. Certainly, people are flawed, and the messages we communicate become less than pure. I wish that shear humility, love, and goodness were in me, but there is indeed also a host of negative and distracting emotions and thoughts, as well. Fortunately, God uses imperfect human beings. All things can be for the good for those who choose to love the Lord and be used according to His purposes.

I believe that God helps us understand things, according to His will for our lives. As my mind began to change, I realized that a person's immune system is healthier without vaccinations for two main reasons. First, a person's immune system is meant to fight disease from the inside out, and harm can result from an injected vaccine.[97] Many complications may arise when the natural path to wellness is interfered with. As Dr.

---

97   "Your Immune System, How It Works And How Vaccines Damage It,"
http://www.vaccineriskawareness.com/your-immune-system-how-it-works-and-how-vaccines-damage-it,
Vaccine Awareness Network, 19 Feb. 2015, web, 03 June 2015.

Richard Moskowitz[98] argues, life is a miracle and cannot be maintained by techno medicine:

> The myth that we can find purely technical solutions to all human ailments seems attractive at first, because it bypasses the problem of healing, which is a genuine miracle in the sense that it can always fail to occur. We are all authentically at risk of illness and death at every moment: no amount of technology can change that. Yet the quixotic mission of techno medicine is precisely to change that: to stand at all times in the front line against disease, to attack and destroy it whenever and wherever it shows itself.

> That is why, with all due respect, I cannot have faith in the miracles or accept the sacraments of Merck, Sharp, and Dohme and the Centers for Disease Control. I prefer to stay with the miracle of life itself, which has given us illness and disease, to be sure, but also the arts of medicine and healing, through which we can acknowledge and experience our pain and vulnerability, and sometimes, with the grace of God and the help of our friends and neighbors, an awareness of health and well-being that knows no boundaries. That is my religion; and while I would willingly share it, I would not force it on anyone.

Second, vaccines change the symbiosis of nature and disease. Jim West writes:

> The word 'virus' is ancient Latin, meaning 'slime' or 'poison.' Mainstream science admits that most viruses are harmless, yet the word 'virus' adds to a biased and highly promoted language of fear regarding nature. Definitions of viruses range from 'pathogenic' to 'not usually pathogenic.' The more popular the media source, the more frightening the definition. Less fearful definitions would change the relationship between the medical industry and its 'patients.' Paradoxically, early virus studies considered virus filtrates to be a poison, not a microbe, thus the name virus. Today, we know that viruses are information.

West continues, commenting on the irony of medical procedures such as chemotherapy, radiation therapy, and the toxic pharmaceuticals "accelerate genetic recombination and thus the potential for a necessary virus proliferation." We seem to have traded the natural order of disease for much nastier and more prevalent situations of cancers and brain damage. With clean water, food with vitamins and nutrients, and simple hygiene, most can be well. Science shows that when this is the case, there are low disease mortality rates.[99] Though diseases may occur, current western nutrition and

---

98   Moskowitz, Richard, MD, "The Case Against Immunizations,"
http://healthimpactnews.com/2015/richard-moskowitz-m-d-the-case-against-immunizations/, Natural Impact News, 27 Feb., 2015, web, 01 June 2015.
99   "Two Centuries of Official Statistics: Proof that Vaccines Did NOT Save Us!,"
http://humansarefree.com/2014/02/2-centuries-of-official-statistics.html?m=0, Humans are Free, 18 Feb. 2014, web, 01 Oct. 2015.

sanitation virtually eliminates serious complications. Each vaccine and disease is particular and should be investigated in order for one to understand the risks. However, as a whole, there is greater risk from current vaccines than from acquiring diseases in nature. The goal is a strong immune system that is able to thrive. Nurturing balance and proper immune system response is our best bet against diseases and even cancer, so prevalent today. It is a way of perceiving wellness, and it deserves our attention right now when even vaccines for cancer are in the works. I think it is essential to realize that the body cannot be made strong and healthy by vaccines, whatever else one believes about their ability to render us immune or not. A strong body is whole and tended holistically, and society deserves health care to consider ways to help us to these ends because many illnesses today are at unprecedented highs.[100]

On a discussion forum on Facebook, the following questions were posted as essential to expose the myths that those in favor of vaccines claim as facts. The following questions were attributed to Del Sharp of "Prevent Disease" and provide a good overview to the missing answers that convince me that the risks of vaccines far outweigh what we have been led to believe are the benefits:

Since the flu pandemic was declared, there have been several so-called 'vaccine experts' coming out of the wood work attempting to justify the effectiveness of vaccines. All of them parrot the same ridiculous historical and pseudoscientific perspectives of vaccinations, which are easily squelched with the following nine questions.

Claim: The study of vaccines, their historical record of achievements, effectiveness, safety and mechanism in humans are well understood and proven in scientific and medical circles.

Fact: The claim is completely false.

1. What to ask: Could you please provide one double blind, placebo-controlled study that can prove the safety and effectiveness of vaccines?

2. What to ask: Could you please provide scientific evidence on ANY study, which can confirm the long-term safety and effectiveness of vaccines?

3. What to ask: Could you please provide scientific evidence, which can prove that disease reduction in any part of the world, at any point in history was attributable to inoculation of populations?

4. What to ask: Could you please explain how the safety and mechanism of vaccines in

100 Cantwell, Alan Jr., M.D., "Are Vaccines Causing More Diseases Than They are Curing," http://www.newdawnmagazine.com/Article/Are_Vaccines_Causing_More_Disease_Than_They_are_Curing.html, New Dawn Magazine, 2,000, web, 09 Sept. 2015.

the human body are scientifically proven if their pharmacokinetics (the study of bodily absorption, distribution, metabolism and excretion of ingredients) are never examined or analyzed in any vaccine study?

One of the most critical elements, which define the toxicity potential of any vaccine, is its pharmacokinetic properties. Drug companies and health agencies refuse to consider the study, analysis or evaluation of the pharmacokinetic properties of any vaccine.

There is not one double blind, placebo-controlled study in the history of vaccine development that has ever proven their safety, effectiveness or achievements (unless those achievements have underlined their damage to human health).

There are also no controlled studies completed in any country, which have objectively proven that vaccines have had any direct or consequential effect on the reduction of any type of disease in any part of the world.

Every single study that has ever attempted to validate the safety and effectiveness of vaccines has conclusively established carcinogenic, mutagenic, and neurotoxic or fertility impairments, but they won't address those.

Claim: Preservatives and chemical additives used in the manufacture of vaccines are safe and no studies have been linked or proven them unsafe for use in humans.

Fact: The claim is completely false.

5. What to ask: Could you please provide scientific justification as to how injecting a human being with a confirmed neurotoxin is beneficial to human health and prevents disease?

6. What to ask: Can you provide a risk/benefit profile on how the benefits of injecting a known neurotoxin exceed its risks to human health for the intended goal of preventing disease?

This issue is no longer even open to debate. It is a scientifically established fact in literally hundreds of studies that the preservatives and chemical additives in vaccines damage cells. Neurotoxicity, immune suppression, immune-mediated chronic inflammation and carcinogenic proliferation are just a few of several effects that have been observed on the human body. See a list of chemicals in vaccines. Fortunately, the drug companies still tell us the damage vaccines have on the human body. People just don't read them. All you have to do is look at the insert for any vaccine, and it will detail the exact ingredients, alerts and potentially lethal effects.

Any medical professional who believes that it is justified to inject any type of neurotoxin into any person to prevent any disease is completely misguided, misinformed, deluded and ignorant of any logic regarding human health.

Claim: Once an individual is injected with the foreign antigen in the vaccine, that individual becomes immune to future infections.

Fact: The claim is completely false.

7. What to ask: Could you please provide scientific justification on how bypassing the respiratory tract (or mucous membrane) is advantageous and how directly injecting viruses into deep muscle tissue enhances immune functioning and prevents future infections?

8. What to ask: Could you please provide scientific justification on how a vaccine would prevent viruses from mutating?

9. What to ask: Could you please provide scientific justification as to how a vaccination can target a virus in an infected individual who does not have the exact viral configuration or strain the vaccine was developed for?

All promoters of vaccination fail to realize that the respiratory tract of humans (actually all mammals) contains antibodies, which initiates natural immune responses within the respiratory tract mucosa. Bypassing this mucosal aspect of the immune system by directly injecting viruses into the muscle (which is vascularized and will enter the blood) leads to a corruption in the immune system itself. As a result, the pathogenic viruses or bacteria cannot be eliminated by the immune system and remain in the body, where they will further grow and/or mutate as the individual is exposed to ever more antigens and toxins in the environment which continue to assault the immune system.

Despite the injection of any type of vaccine, viruses continue circulating through the body, mutating and transforming into other organisms. The ability of a vaccine manufacturer to target the exact viral strain without knowing its mutagenic properties is equivalent to shooting a gun at a fixed target that has already been moved from its location. You would be shooting at what was, not what is!

Flu viruses, may mutate, change or adapt several times over a period of one flu season, making the seasonal influenza vaccine 100% redundant and ineffective every single flu season. Ironically, the natural immune defenses of the human body can target these changes but the vaccines cannot.

I have never encountered one pro-vaccine advocate, whether medically or scientifically qualified, who could answer even one let alone all nine of these questions. One or all of the following will happen when debating any of the above questions:

They will concede defeat and admit they are stumped.

They will attempt to discredit unrelated issues that do not pertain to the question.

They will formulate their response and rebuttal based on historical arguments and scientific studies, which have been disproved repeatedly.

Not one pro-vaccine advocate will ever directly address these questions in an open mainstream venue.

No one wants to believe that vaccination is harmful, or to move through the depth of the rabbit hole once it can't be denied. No one wants to experience social isolation, regret for harm that a vaccine may have caused, or to distrust doctors' claims. However, I value living whole, and am called to live holy. I am willing to seek Truth with faith in God. Good can increase in this world with my humble efforts. Picking up my Cross and following Christ preserves my life and others', even though losing it is inevitable.

CHAPTER 3

The Right to Life: Diseases Today and False Herd Immunity

Further on, this chapter examines the prevalence of illnesses today among children and the incorrect assumption that vaccinations provide "herd immunity." To begin, my belief is that vaccination must not be mandated because people deserve the right to preserve the sanctity of life in wholeness and holiness.

As we sent our daughter to preschool, I was in the throes of researching the snot out of vaccination. Ohio did not yet mandate vaccination, and with a statement that we were not placing our daughter (or others) in harm by exempting her from vaccines, which we believed were not in her best interest, and a legal exemption form, our daughter was able to attend school.

It was a sign of our times, but no less shocking, when I received an email from our local school district concerning my boys who were enrolled in grades three and five. The subject was "Immunization Records," with a message following that misled parents to believe that vaccinations were already mandatory for school attendance:

> Attention all ... parents: State law requires all students to be up-to-date on their immunizations in order to attend school. <u>Per Ohio Revised Code 3313.671 (Section A, 2) students should be excluded from school after 14 days of school if shot records are not provided to the school.</u> *All required shot records for your child need to be turned in to the school clinic or your child will be excluded from school starting Monday, September 21, 2015.* For all Kindergarten parents, please be sure all information has been received by your school clinic as many shot records have not been received. For all 7th-grade parents, please be sure your child has had his/her T-dap booster and records for this are turned in to the ... clinic BEFORE September 21, 2015. If you have already provided this information to your school, thank you, and please disregard this email.
>
> Please call your primary physician or the County Health Department for an appointment. The County Health Department has walk-in clinics available and they can be reached at XXX-XXX-XXXX.

The school district's email followed protocol set in motion by the state, and it frightened me that the school would omit the important second half of the law on reasons for exemption. The school district's message was based on the law: "3313.671 [Effective Until 10/15/2015] Proof of required immunizations – exceptions." Currently in the state of Ohio, a student has a right to exemption for five reasons including having had the natural disease(s), reasons of conscience (including religious convictions), and in cases where a physician considers the vaccine medically contraindicated.

All the way back in 1999, the Association of American Physicians and Surgeons stated:

> Public policy regarding vaccines is fundamentally flawed. It is permeated by conflicts of interest. It is based on poor scientific methodology (including studies that are too small, too short, and too limited in populations represented), which is, moreover, insulated from independent criticism. The evidence is far too poor to warrant overriding the independent judgments of patients, parents, and attending physicians, even if this were ethically or legally acceptable. Indeed, evidence is accumulating that serious adverse reactions are being ignored. [For example ....] [F]or most children, the risk of a serious vaccine reaction may be 100 times greater than the risk of hepatitis B.[101]

Americans should not mandate vaccination for reasons Catherine Diodati, spokesperson for Vaccine Choice Canada, argues. She claims vaccines pose risks and each individual deserves adequate disclosure prior to providing consent.[102]

> In order to provide truly informed consent, individuals must be apprised of potential risks, benefits and alternatives to vaccination. Pertinent information should include the actual risk of contracting a particular disease, based upon epidemiological evidence, probable outcome and available treatments. Disclosure should also include vaccine ingredients and their known hazards, possible adverse effects and vaccine efficacy.

Diodati argues that vaccination consent should be based upon accurate and adequate disclosure and not upon fear, such as the mass email from our school district, or countless horror stories of doctors telling people that they will die without the vaccine, and that the probable outcome of natural infection should be explained. She claims patients should be informed of proper nutrition and vitamins.

She argues for a consent process to include information on the legal status of vaccination recommendations as well as the types of, and how to obtain, exemptions.

> Where mandatory vaccination legislation does not exist, individuals clearly should be informed that vaccination is voluntary. In regions where vaccination legislation does exist, thorough information regarding exemptions should be made available prior to obtaining consent. While medical exemptions do carry

101 Orient, Dr. Jane M., "Mandating Vaccines: Government Practicing Medicine Without a License?," The Medical Sentinel, 4 no.5 (1999): 166-168.
102 Diodati, Catherine, "Policy Statement on Vaccination," http://vaccinechoicecanada.com/about/policy-statement-on-vaccination/, Vaccine Choice Canada (formerly VRAN), 2015, web, 05 July 2015.

certain limitations, patients, and their parents or guardians, should be informed that religious and philosophical exemptions carry no such limitations. Exemption forms, where required, should be readily available.

Diodati claims that there should be no pressure exerted to gain vaccination compliance, and children are only removed from a school setting for the duration of an outbreak, and only if the child is not already immune. "At no time should any coercion be exerted to influence a vaccination decision. Neither social service payments, medical treatment, employment, professional standing, nor the patient-care provider relationship, should be threatened based upon vaccination status."

She continues in her statement outlining vaccine recommendations, which continue to be expanded, "despite a lack of supporting evidence demonstrating need, safety, or efficacy." The community and its physicians did not agree there was a danger sufficient to justify the development of hepatitis B and varicella universal vaccination recommendations, or the flu shot recommendation. (In fact, she sites studies that show giving the flu shot to children worsens their respiratory system.) The varicella vaccination for chickenpox, an innocuous disease for healthy children, has been developed, along with a heightened fear of the disease, at astronomical cost. The vaccine "carries the risk of altering the disease's epidemiology by deferring the disease to adolescence or adulthood, when the disease is more severe." Not to mention the fact that the chickenpox vaccine sheds, and my non-vaccinated daughters got the virus from one who was shedding after vaccination. Of course, I am happy, considering my girls had a few pox, were mildly warm, and after three days, there was hardly a sign of the infection. This is nature's way, when children are healthy and young. Vaccinating all children for hepatitis B is unnecessary, impractical, and dangerous. Diodati explains the low risk of the disease as merely three percent of 3,000 cases of natural hepatitis B for children, and immunity to hepatitis B has not been shown to persist to adulthood.

Vaccines should not be mandatory because of the risks associated with vaccination, as Diodati notes.

Vaccines are inherently hazardous products, which contain attenuated live, or inactivated, antigens, germicides, detergents, preservatives, adjuvants, and residues from culture media and host tissues. Vaccine manufacturers are allowed a certain amount of competitive secrecy regarding the formulation of vaccines. While this protects the manufacturer's competitive edge, it neither protects vaccine recipients nor facilitates the informed consent process. Many vaccines contain formaldehyde as a disinfectant. Formaldehyde is not only carcinogenic but it is known to be unpredictable as a disinfectant, sometimes causing antigenic proteins to clump, hardening the outer gelatinous debris, which is digested by the body allowing fully virulent particles to be released in the vaccine. Other vaccine chemicals are equally toxic and can cause cumulative and long-term adverse effects on the body. For example, phenol is a highly caustic coal tar derivative used in vaccines. Phenol is a protoplasmic poison (i.e., toxic to all cells), inhibits phagocytic activity (i.e., activity of a cell, such as a white blood cell, that engulfs and absorbs waste material, harmful microorganisms, or other foreign bodies in the bloodstream and tissues), and has been associated with systemic poisoning among other adverse effects. Aluminum salts and gels, used as vaccine adjuvants, have been associated with motor paralysis, fatty degeneration of the kidneys and liver, learning disabilities, dementia, bone dissolution, et cetera.

In addition to the harmful ingredients, she argues that vaccines introduce "novel pathogens, and genetic material, into humans. The result of which may well be the permanent alteration of the human genome and the perpetuation of vaccine-induced degenerative diseases ad infinitum." It is evident that something other than wellness is at stake when the government aims to mandate vaccination at the same time as many new vaccines are under development and this despite the fact that science has failed to identify and remedy risks associated with current vaccines.

Diodati argues for the development of appropriate screening methods to be used prior to the administration of any vaccine. She claims, though there has been compelling evidence linking vaccines to SIDS, autism, diabetes, transverse myelitis, arthritis and many other long-term disabilities, there is no screening method used to determine which individuals will be placed at risk. Her thorough policy statement on vaccination explains why mandatory vaccination harms society.

Statistics from the CDC show one in six children in the U.S. "had a developmental disability in 2006-2008, ranging from mild disabilities such as speech and language impairments to serious developmental disabilities, such as intellectual disabilities, cerebral palsy, and autism."[103] Sadly, families may not think vaccines had anything to do with children's problems. A student recently told me that her brother is autistic, but it wasn't because of the vaccines. She simply suggested, "How could vaccines have changed all that about him. No, he was born that way." I assured her that she and her family know her brother, but vaccines can damage the brain, they can cause it to swell, and so.... I understood in that moment how hard it is to imagine that something we believe is healthy can harm us so desperately, especially when our doctors, the experts, argue there isn't causation between vaccines and brain trauma that causes autism. Even when adults are harmed, after having been healthy, there is often a time period of other diagnoses and sometimes an indefinite period of denial, that vaccination had anything at all to do with the individual's problem(s).

---

103 "CDC | Data and Statistics | Autism Spectrum Disorder (ASD) | NCBDDD," http://www.cdc.gov/ncbdd/autism/data.html, United States Centers for Disease Control and Prevention, 12 Aug. 2015, web, 01 Sept. 2015.

However, parents or caretakers may learn that vaccines cause harm through personal experience following vaccination, and believe that their doctors are missing something. Health care providers do not often explain the harm as being caused by vaccines because most are trained to perceive vaccine harm as an unlikely correlation not a causation supported by science. This is the routine belief, despite scientific research which supports that many of today's disorders are linked to vaccine injury. Those who have studied links between vaccine and injury have argued that food allergies, attention or affective disorders, such as ADHD / ADD and autism, or developmental delays, often in speech and memory, are *caused* by vaccination.

Scientist Judy Mikovits explains that cause means one to one. She says that to argue vaccines cause a problem, every case of giving the vaccine would then result in harm. For example, some are vaccinated and do not become autistic and, therefore, some argue vaccines do not cause autism. As has already been discussed, and as Judy Mikovits argues in the extended YouTube cited above, every time one is vaccinated there is potential for numerous harms that may not be seen even in one's lifetime but that may alter the very genes of a human being. No one who is vaccinated can know if they will be fortunate and dodge the "bullet" or if they, for a number of immune-level reasons, will be harmed. There's currently no test to determine whether a given vaccine is a risk for certain individuals, other than the obvious fact that when one is ill or already diagnosed with an acute disease, one is not supposed to be vaccinated. When a baby is first born, there is little to no chance that parents would know if Heb B would cause a reaction on their baby. When an infant is two months, there is still little chance that it could be known that the child was at risk. In addition, when my boys were slightly under the weather with a cold, the pediatrician still administered the "safe and effective" vaccines. The only thing that seems common knowledge is that those who are ill and cannot be vaccinated must be "protected" by all others who have to be vaccinated to offer this protection. In reality, a sick person is a risk to other persons, and being vaccinated causes less health in all people. Ironic.

For my argument, which is concerned with the rhetoric of vaccination (as I am not a scientist presenting my own conclusive data to show definite results) causation is used when a person believes that data (experience, science, observations of others, etc.) illustrates a link. Correlation is used when a person is skeptical of the link between vaccines and harm. In my research, the more evidence linking autism and vaccines, the more autism seems caused, not merely correlated, with vaccination. The other possible links just don't add up. For example, some argue that autism is genetic, but in Mark Blaxill's article, "Out of Africa and Into Autism,"[104] he discusses how studies among Africans show that autism can be acquired.

---

104 Blaxill, Mark, "Out of Africa and Into Autism: More Evidence Illuminates the Somali Anomaly in Minnesota," http://www.ageofautism.com/2008/11/out-of-africa-a.html, Age of Autism, 24 Nov. 2008, web, 7 Sept. 2015

Blaxill begins with the reminder that autism was once rare in America. It was actually lower here than in other parts of the developed world. Leo Kanner discovered the illness among a small group of kids in the States in the 1930s and conducted a study in the 40s. With some "broad-based environmental exposures," autism rates are up in the U.S. to 1 in 100 children, he claims. Other research indicates autism is even higher in certain groups. The CDC states that 1 in 42 boys has autism, and 1 in 189 girls have autism.[105] In "Out of Africa and Into Autism," Blaxill tells of a Somali community of political refugees in Minnesota acquiring autism, which had been foreign to them before coming to the West and having access to our health care. In another study in the 1980s, African immigrants also showed a high incidence of autism among their newly vaccinated children.

Blaxill makes three main points: autism was always rare in Africa; autism occurred among elite families with access to western health services; and among Africans who migrate to western countries, autism rates are high, and they face unusual risk of over-vaccination. Even among the African people, autism was explained as genetic, but with continued studies, it was noted that after malaria some became autistic. It was then surmised that autism could be acquired, but researchers concluded that if it were a result of malaria, then many more would be autistic. Blaxill states the connection: in addition to malaria infections, the elite children with access to western health care had been vaccinated. Studies among African populations illustrate a high vaccination risk because certain diseases are foreign to these groups of people. Their immune systems are not equipped to protect them from the disease. Blaxill argues:

> The obvious risk that immigrants to any western country, both Sweden and America, face is over vaccination. As vaccination programs have spread around the world in recent years, future immigrants are increasingly likely to be vaccinated in their home countries. When they travel, they are forced to receive another round of vaccinations in their home countries before they leave. When they reach their new countries, their previous vaccination records are generally not recognized as valid and they often must be vaccinated again. This unique migration risk is especially relevant for population groups that can influence autism risk: women of childbearing age, pregnant women and infants. It's hard to know what kind of havoc these redundant treatments wreck on the immune system of such targets when they receive excessive vaccine doses. All we know is that children of modern immigrants are at high risk of both over vaccination and of autism.

It cannot be denied: autism is rare among those who are not vaccinated. Period. World-over. If one understands vaccination may harm individuals, then people who aim

---

105 "CDC | Data and Statistics | Autism Spectrum Disorder (ASD) | NCBDDD," http://www.cdc.gov/ncbdd/autism/data.html, United States Centers for Disease Control and Prevention, 12 Aug. 2015, web, 01 Sept. 2015.

to help those in less developed nations would have to reconsider the ways they offer help. These caring individuals would likely face feelings of remorse, and this is another reason to resist changing one's mind on vaccination. Many in third world countries do not have access to western health care, and those who do, have had less western health care over time. There are plans to push vaccines worldwide, but, interestingly, other countries do not as readily accept vaccines (among other pharmaceuticals).[106]

Importantly, autism is not only a risk for Africans but is a risk for each of us, as the now-called "father of the anti-vaccine movement," British surgeon and medical researcher Dr. Andrew Wakefield found in his studies.[107] In 1998, The Lancet published and retracted Wakefield's report that suggested a link between the MMR vaccine and autism. (Since that time, many other scientific journals published Wakefield's research, though we do not hear of this in the States.)

Wakefield's report showed a problem concerning vaccines and the immune system, which is largely located in the gut. His research added to the concern that thimerosal contributed to the risk for autism because he found that the MMR vaccine harnessed the body's immune system, beginning in the gut, and made that person his own worst enemy. He was banned from practicing medicine for his claims. Wakefield says that he is no longer a part of the system that would have him fall in line and obey orders that ultimately come from pharmaceutical companies "and others." He says that he is free, and in his freedom, he is stepping up and out to lead others against mandatory vaccination bills. Autism rates are at all-time highs in the U.S. for all children, and this deserves our careful attention, particularly in regards to vaccination, as there is a variety of evidence supporting causation.

Some argue there is no scientific evidence supporting the link between autism and vaccination. They claim that Dr. Wakefield's report way back in the late 1990's was proven wrong. Yet, there are over 30 scientific studies (over 49 on the Internet) linking autism and vaccination.[108] Even President Obama, before he was elected, stated concern that vaccination caused autism. After assuming office and establishing Obamacare, heavily funded by pharmaceutical companies, he no longer discusses this growing problem.[109]

---

106 Xiao, Kaijing, "Glaxosmithkline Fined $488.8M for 'Massive Bribery Network'," http://abcnews.go.com/International/glaxosmithkline-gsk-fined-4888-million-massive-bribery-network/story?id=25624684, Abc News, 19 Sept. 2014, web, 20 Sept. 2015.
107 Rebecca Plevin, "Discredited Vaccination Opponent Andrew Wakefield Crusades Against California SB 277 | 89.3 KPCC," http://www.scpr.org/news/2015/05/01/51367/discredited-vaccination-opponent-andrew-wakefield/, Southern California Public Radio, 01 May 2015, web, 04 June 2015.
108 Goes, Lisa Joyce, "30 Scientific Studies Showing the Link between Vaccines and Autism," http://www.whale.to/v/30_scientific_studies.html, May 2015, web, 01 Sept. 2015.
109 "Obama 'Skyrocketing Autism Rate' From Vaccines," http://edgytruth.com/2015/09/21/obama-skyrocketing-autism-rate-from-vaccines/, 21 Sept. 2015, web, 01 Oct. 2015.

In fact, autism has been proven to be on a drastic incline that parallels vaccination, beginning with Leo Kanner's study in the 1940's of 11 children who first illustrated what had been very unusual affective disorder, which has been named "autism." At this point in history, the smallpox vaccine was administered using thimerosal. In Lisa Goes's article, she argues that parents who believe their child's risk of brain injury from vaccination is higher than their risk from disease have the right to decline vaccination. There is ample evidence to support this claim. She also argues that parents often know more about potential vaccine risks than top public officials.

The theories that autism is genetic and that the characterization of autism is too inclusive and variable to be useful in clinical studies is not persuasive to me in light of increased amounts of the toxic thimerosal preservative injected into vaccinated children. Rev. Lisa Sykes cites studies[110] on vaccine ingredients showing that the toxic preservative, thimerosal, is in fact still used, and more thimerosal is injected into children today than in 1999 when it was first declared unsafe. The flu shots have increased levels of thimerosal to the degree that is only safe for one who weighs 550 lbs. She presents studies that also show the genes of girls and boys with autism reveal the impossibility of a genetic correlate to autism. So far, Rev. Sykes is the only article I have read from a church leader calling a Christian community to a "bold witness against vaccine manufacturers" because of the harm of vaccines as they are currently being used. Her position differs from the one in this book because she does not get into the fact that fetal stem cells are used in vaccine production, and at the end, she argues that their position is not entirely anti-vaccine.

My argument is predicated upon the Orthodox Christian understanding of personhood: body and spirit. Based on the Faith, my belief is that becoming whole is preserving the sanctity of life by living whole and holy. I agree with her, and the Methodist community with whom she worships, and argue for safety and informed consent. It seems to me that vaccination by nature of its history and current practice cannot be safe and therefore we will not be informed (because we would never agree if we knew the risk). This is why I am anti-vaccine.

I have experience with autistic children, and their behavior is striking; it is not merely over-diagnosed. There is a beautiful mother at church with a grown daughter who is autistic. The daughter, now a young woman, comes to Liturgy once a month and receives Holy Communion after the rest of us have left the sanctuary. She cannot handle the noise and confusion of the many parishioners, though she knows many details of our lives, embraces me with great bear-hugs, and is full of love and life. Her mother says that she is a gift, always has been, and thanks God for the daughter who will always need her mother because she is, developmentally, three years old.

110 Sykes, Rev. Lisa K., "TEN LIES Told by Those Who Say 'Mercury in Vaccines is Safe: Refuted by a Mother who Knows Better," *Trace Amounts – the documentary on mercury and its role in the autism epidemic*, http://traceamounts.com/ten-lies-told-about-mercury-in-vaccines/, Sept. 2015, web, 19 Sept. 2015.

Certainly, each child is a gift from God, and having autism does not change that. God, the Giver of Life, the Lord, does not make us ill, and in His great and perfect love, He suffers with us in this fallen world. A father defended his son with autism, saying that the Creator made his son with autism. It made me very sad. I respect this father's ability to let go of anger and blame. Yet, it is important to realize that God does not will for us to be ill or to die. This is a reality of a fallen world that is riddled by sins that we are called to fight, even as we must also pick up our crosses and follow after Him, enduring all things in love and hope. God allows our struggles, but, in the case of vaccination, we can prevent some harm, if we know the risk and understand that we can build our bodies stronger without vaccines. The wages of sin are death, and there is no escape this side of eternity. The Orthodox Christian teaching is that the fall, through sin, makes what was to be perfect, broken. People are to love in all circumstances, but illness, death, and evil is not meant to be considered good or the way God made us to be.

Environmental toxicity is linked to autism. Toxic chemicals on food and seeds contribute to our bodies' toxic overloads. A Senior Research Scientist at MIT, Stephanie Seneff, who spent three decades of her life researching biology and technology, with a current focus on nutrition and health, argued that half of all children in the States would be autistic by 2025, if the rate of autism continues to increase as it is.[111] She is anti-vaccine and anti-GMO, and her research on autism demonstrates a remarkably consistent correlation between the use of Roundup on crops and GMO seeds and rising rates of autism. Many are alarmed by the fact that reprogrammed insect virus, as a genetically modified organism, is now used in some flu shots. (GM mosquitos have been developed and released into the wild as a protective measure against malaria.) The flu shot using GMOs has been on the market since 2014[112], even though two people actually died when the vaccine was tested, before hitting the market.[113] GM vaccines[114] are argued cheap and "safe" alternatives to traditional vaccines, and GM hepatitis B vaccines are currently in the works. In addition, edible GM vaccines, which would be absorbed into the bloodstream when eaten, are alternatives for less developed countries without the necessary refrigeration and sterile needles. Such vaccines are in development for HIV/AIDS, TB, cancer, among other diseases. We do not know the ramifications of such vaccines, but considering the problems we currently face in our society's health, I do not support the plan to further the vaccination program using

---

111 "Half of all Children will be Autistic by 2025, Warns Senior Research Scientist at MIT," http://www.anh-usa.org/half-of-all-children-will-be-autistic-by-2025-warns-senior-research-scientist-at-mit/, Alliance for Natural Health USA: Good Science and Good Law, 23 Dec. 2014, web, 01 Sept. 2015.
112 Walia, Arjun, "FDA Approves First GMO Flu Vaccine: Expected on Market in 2014," http://www.collective-evolution.com/2013/07/12/fda-approves-first-gmo-flu-vaccine-expected-on-market-in-2014/, Collective Evolution, 12 July 2013, web, 05 July 2015.
113 Mercola, Dr. Joseph, "Are You Concerned over Genetically Modified Vaccines," http://www.nvic.org/NVIC-vaccine-news/October-2012/Are-You-Concerned-Over-Genetically-Modified-Vaccin.aspx, National Vaccine Information Center, 02 Oct. 2012, web, 01 Sept. 2015.
114 Diaz, Julia, "GMOs in Medicine and Research," http://www.britannica.com/science/genetically-modified-organism, Encyclopedia Britannica, Inc., 24 Aug. 2015, web, 01 Oct. 2015.

GM/GMO vaccines.[115]

My scientist friend said that "evidence based science / Medicine", agrees that there is a link between environmental toxicity and heavy metal contamination, but extending this to vaccines is circumstantial. Considering the above information, and much more below, I disagree. We agree that thimerosal is "no good," and he says that is why "there are thimerosal-free formulations." The problem is that few are offered vaccines without the preservative, and the lax safety checks on current and future vaccines poses a great challenge to all of us. He argues that dihydrogen oxide provides 100% correlation as a toxic environmental agent. To which I reply, "Yes, my friend. You are the scientist, but sipping my coffee from Styrofoam is not injecting thimerosal into the deep muscle tissue (which would enter the bloodstream) of a pregnant mother, infant, or developing child." It seems obvious that vaccines provide the link to environmental toxicity and neural impairment. No other substance is as ubiquitous and constant, and few other neurotoxins are injected into our children.

Children receive the majority of vaccines, and with immature immune systems, they are more likely to experience harm. Still, vaccines can harm, and even kill, adults. A friend was re-vaccinated in her late twenties when moving from Canada to the States. She developed mental and physical problems so desperate that doctors diagnosed her with degenerative disorders such as multiple sclerosis. After unraveling her health issues, she learned that she had autoimmune disease. Later, she was diagnosed with ovarian cancer. She had been in favor of vaccines until her health declined so rapidly after re-vaccination as an adult. Now, with her two sons also vaccinated, and also with autoimmune disease, she uses food, herbs, and oils to heal herself and her family. If vaccines were mandated, she and her children could die. Mandatory vaccination threatens to limit medical exemptions[116] for almost all individuals. However, most states continue to have available exemptions[117], contrary to the mainstream suggestion that non-vaccinated children cannot attend school in states where vaccines are mandatory. Because fewer would push against the "rule," if vaccination were mandated, many more adults would become ill with autoimmune disorders, allergies and intolerances.

Deaths often go unexplained after vaccinations. A healthy fifteen-month-old girl had her year-old pictures taken with her beautiful family. They wore jeans and white t-shirts, all with dark hair and healthy glowing skin. The child was loving and eager to bond with others, and even the photographer received her kisses. The girl had two older brothers

115 Brogan, Kelly MD, "Connecting the Dots: GMOs and Vaccines," http://www.greenmedinfo.com/blog/connecting-dots-gmos-and-vaccines, GreenMedInfo, 12 Nov. 2013, web, 01 Oct. 2015.
116 Feller, Stephen, "AMA Supports Tighter Limit on Non-Medical Vaccine Exemptions," http://www.upi.com/Health_News/2015/06/10/AMA-supports-tighter-limit-on-non-medical-vaccine-exemptions/5011433938054, 10 June 2015, web, 20 July 2015.
117 Tietje, Kate, "No Shots, No School, Not True," http://www.modernalternativemama.com/2012/09/15/no-shots-no-school-not-true/, Modern Alternative Momma, 10 Oct. 2015, web, 10 Oct. 2015.

who took turns holding her, their parents smiling in the background. At the baby's year-old doctor's appointment, she was vaccinated. There was nothing remarkable afterwards, just a slight fever and "normal" fussiness post-vaccination. The next morning, when mom went to get the baby who seemed to be sleeping, the child was dead. Upon autopsy results, there was no cause, and the baby was pronounced SUDC (Sudden Unexplained Death in Childhood). Even delaying vaccinations, as this family did, can result in much regret. Unexplained infant deaths have increased with the introduction of vaccines.[118]

In my experience, those most resistant to reconsideration of current medical practices are those whose lives have been dedicated to health care, both patients (who have had health issues and relied on care) and medical professionals. That is, unless one has directly seen and or experienced illness and or death as a result of current medical practices. A friend has a daughter with special needs. Her autoimmune disease makes her highly susceptible to disease and illness. The mother had been leery of vaccinations but with the extreme push of the child's doctors, she and her family have been vaccinated. The whole family receives the annual flu shot; they want to "cover all of their bases because her health continues to worsen." (I wonder if the family considers that the worsening health may be a result of the approach to her care.) The child has a folder of health conditions that continues to grow thicker, and she even has to wear a helmet to protect her from falling because she could die from the injury or infection. When things are not increasing our own health, or the health of our children, we should try something different, even if it means re-considering the entire approach to our wellness. With the child's extremely vulnerable condition, communicable diseases pose a grave danger, but there are safer alternatives to vaccines, such as homeoprophlaxis.[119] Several studies have demonstrated HP to be as effective as conventional vaccination, but without the toxicity. In her blog, Dr. Levatin explains:

HP has been used for more than 200 years. It is similar to conventional vaccination, in the sense that it introduces small doses of pathogens (bacteria and viruses) to 'train' the immune system to respond effectively if an active pathogen is encountered. However, instead of injecting bits of bacteria, inactivated viruses and other toxic ingredients, HP utilizes homeopathic nosodes given orally. Nosodes are specially prepared diluted and succussed (agitated) preparations of infectious agents. They are so diluted that they no longer contain any measurable amounts of the actual microbes; all that remains is their energetic frequencies. Unlike vaccines, nosodes are completely safe, and gently train the immune system to learn how to respond appropriately, when the treated person is exposed to microbes that could cause an illness.

118 Scheibner, Dr. Viera, *Vaccination: 100 Years of Orthodox Research shows that Vaccines Represent a Medical Assault on the Immune System*, Co-Creative Designs, 1993.
119 Levatin, Janet MD, "Homeoprophlaxis: A Nontoxic Alternative for Promoting Wellness," http://tenpennyimc.com/2013/08/07/homeoprophlaxis-a-nontoxic-alternative-to-staying-well/, Tenpenny IMC, 07 Aug. 2013, web, 01 Sept. 2015.

Despite the cases of reported paralysis and even death, new vaccines continue on the market. For example, the HPV vaccination is currently administered to teenaged boys and girls under the claim that the vaccine can protect one from cancer and genital warts, though even the CDC has taken a closer look at Gardasil and its dangers in recent years.[120] Five years ago, the insert for the vaccine indicated that it was not for boys, and we have yet to learn what the long-term effects may be on boys (and girls) who are vaccinated with HPV. The most frightening aspect of the current vaccination program is that even though children are suffering extreme nerve damage after vaccination with HPV, and even though this vaccine is not needed, good-intentioned doctors advise patients to vaccinate. Even more disturbing, there is a current push to mandate the HPV vaccine, though HPV is not a communicable disease. Parents of teenagers in Indiana who refused the HPV vaccine were sent a letter from the state.[121] "There is absolutely no proof that these vaccines work at all, yet there is a great deal of evidence that they cause lifelong injuries to those teens who do take them. Yet now, in order to increase distribution and revenue, the suggestion is to push them to the infant market."[122]

More vaccines do not equal more well. The government and CDC are tied to pharmaceutical companies through money, rather than a common goal to make Americans well. Vaccinations harm the body's natural immune system, and there is hard science to prove it. "Big Pharma" and "Big Food" corporations donate large sums of money to health care providers and medical schools for their research to be uncontested. The favorable results of studies financially supported by these organizations become scientific evidence to prove vaccines (and other drugs) are safe, effective, and beneficial. Those who question the effects of vaccines, often observing the harm first hand and then researching vaccine risks, are written off because there would be a loss of billions of dollars and because vaccination is simply accepted practice. Pharmaceutical companies pour money into educational training of health care providers. They advertise directly to heath care providers, and even though strong-willed doctors say that the pharmaceutical companies do not persuade them, when patients have needs, as a commercial's jingle in the mind of a patient, is the pharmaceutical representative's pitch in the mind of a doctor. Even for doctors who have absolutely no contact with pharmaceutical reps, the medical community is not immune to the persuasion. As a collective, vaccines continue to be considered essential against communicable diseases that kill people. It is a strange thing, considering most of these diseases are not a threat when one is healthy. It is strange to me that doctors wouldn't push harder for patients to simply get healthier, overall. On the one hand, people are

---

120 Kotz, Deborah, "CDC Takes Closer Look at Gardasil and Paralysis," http://health.usnews.com/health-news/blogs/on-women/2009/03/20/cdc-takes-closer-look-at-gradasil-and-paralysis, U.S. News and World Report, 20 Mar. 2009, web, 01 Sept. 2015.
121 "Indiana Sends Letters to Parents of Unvaccinated Children," http://vaxxtercom/index.php/2015/10/21/indiana-sends-letters-to-parents-of-unvaccinated-children/, Vaxxter: Anti-Vaccination News, 21 Oct. 2015, web, 21 Oct. 2015.
122 "HPV Vaccination for Infants. It's Coming.," http://edgytruth.com/2015/07/15/hpv-vaccination-for-infants-be-worried, Edgy Truth, 15 July 2015, web, 10 Aug. 2015.

losing trust in doctors who seem ever ready to prescribe a medication instead of getting to the source of one's illness, but on the other hand, there is an increasing reliance on doctors and prescriptions. In Catherine Diodati's policy statement for Vaccine Choice Canada argues public confidence in health care is low:

> Public-trust in pharmaceutical companies has diminished severely. Public confidence in government and health officials has eroded. While vaccine manufacturers were once perceived to be altruistic in intent, they continue to lose public confidence through the release of unnecessarily dangerous and expensive products, unsupported claims regarding safety, efficacy and need, persecution of researchers whose results do not support the use of their products, inadequate and contaminated production lines, and market manipulation.

She provides illustrations of pharmaceutical companies profiting at the cost of our health. In 2,000, the flu vaccine went from $30.00 a vial to $100.00. An anthrax vaccine was known to be contaminated but was given anyways to military in the U.S. and Canada. If one refused, there was a good chance of court marshal and or discharge. Diadoti explains that rotavirus is not a threat in the U.S., as it is in other countries, as children have clean water and more nutrition available to them. The vaccine companies sell the rotavirus vaccine at lower rates to poorer nations, with the agreement that the U.S. will purchase the vaccine in bulk at a higher rate. All of our babies are given a vaccine that is unnecessary. With this in mind, I cringe with the argument that science proves the effectiveness of vaccination because, in truth, science supports the claims of need and safety that the pharmaceutical companies want the rest of us to buy.

Many childhood diseases that one is vaccinated against are not life threatening, even if they are contracted. The body can naturally recover and build life-long immunity from having many diseases, which is often—if not always—preferable to autism, anaphylaxis, or encephalitis. Some argue these are infrequent reactions, but the risks do not outweigh the benefits because the risks are severe, and they are indeed more frequent than we are told. Ultimately, there is no point in vaccinations because they do not protect one from disease.

Dr. Tetyana Obukhanych argues vaccines are the basis of allergies, not immunization. She also claims that vaccines destroy natural immunity, which is the basis for true "herd immunity."[123] She points to the limitations of preventing childhood diseases by short-term "protective effects of live attenuated viral vaccines" that leave mothers without immunity for their infants, should exposure occur. She argues that vaccination disrupts disease transmission, and reduces the chances of exposure, "rather than establishing a population's immunity. By doing so, vaccination campaigns wipe out population's

---

123 "Dr. Tetyana Obukhanych: The Myth of Herd Immunity," http://vaccine-injury.info/tetyana.cfm, Vaccine Injury Info., 2015, web, 05 Oct. 2015.

immunity to childhood diseases rather than help to maintain it." In the past, when diseases were immune in adult populations through naturally occurring immunity after infection, then mothers passed this immunity to breastfed infants.

Many mothers today deal with guilt because our kids are ill, and we don't know why. The peanut allergy is an epidemic that has resulted from the combination of vaccines currently administered to infants, according to Heather Fraser[124] and Dr. Tim O'Shea[125], among others[126]. She explains how peanut allergic mice are created in a lab when mice eat or are forced to inhale peanut protein fused to a bacterial toxin like diphtheria or cholera. The Hib vaccine is similar to the peanut protein on a molecular level, she argues. Because the body confuses the two, an allergy to peanut can often result. In the 1800s, Dr. Clemens Von Pirquet coined the word "allergy." He was a leading researcher of the new disease "serum sickness," which resulted from the first mass allergic phenomenon in history as a result of the introduction of the hypodermic needle. He noted then that injecting intact proteins into the blood would create a sort of immunity along with hypersensitivity, or allergy. In the early 1900s, many doctors were against vaccines for this reason.

Many children have allergies, and we have been told that this has nothing to do with vaccinations. According to Barbara Feick Gregory, "the main cause of all food allergies is vaccinations and injections and the secondary cause is antibiotics and other drugs."[127] The peanut allergy in particular is directly caused by the current vaccination program because peanut oil has been used (and continues to be used) in vaccines, including the influenza vaccine and the vitamin K shot, since the 1960s, according to Dr. Palevsky[128], among others.[129] The vitamin K shot immediately administered to newborns is not necessary and can be harmful, according to Dr. Cees Vermeer who was interviewed by Dr. Mercola.[130] It is argued that many newborns are deficient and need vitamin K for necessary blood clotting, but they can receive sufficient vitamin K from their mother by not cutting the umbilical cord for the first five minutes of life. The shot presents risks

---

124 Fraser, Heather, *The Peanut Allergy Epidemic: What's Causing it and How to Stop it*, Skyhorse Publishing, 2011.
125 O' Shea, Dr. Tim, "Vaccines and the Peanut Allergy Epidemic,"
http://www.thedoctorwithin.com/allergies/vaccines-and-the-peanut-allergy-epidemic/, MMXV The Doctor Within, 2015, web, 01 Oct. 2015.
126 "How to Cause a Peanut Allergy Epidemic in 4 Easy Steps," http://thinkingmomsrevolution.com/whats-really-behind-peanut-allergy-epidemic/, The Thinking Moms' Revolution, 18 Aug. 2015, web, 01 Sept. 2015.
127 Feick, Barbara, "Vaccinations are the MAIN CAUSE of Food Allergies," http://barbfeick.com/vaccinations/, 2009, web, 01 April 2015.
128 Palevsky, Dr. Lawrence, "Peanut Oil Used in Vaccines Since the 1960s,"
http://www.drpalevsky.com/articles_pages/346_peanut_oil_in_vaccines_since%20the_1960s.asp, 2011, web, 01 Oct. 2015.
129 Ring, J., et al., "Allergy to Peanut Oil—Clinically Relevant?,"
http://www.ncbi.nlm.nih.gov/m/pubmed/17373969, PubMed, 2007, web, 05 Sept. 2015.
130 Mercola, Dr. Joseph, "The Potential Dark Side of the Routine Newborn Vitamin K Shot,"
http://articles.mercola.com/sites/articles/archive/2010/03/27/high-risks-to-your-baby-from-vitamin-k-shot-they-dont-warn-you-about.aspx, Mercola, 3 March 2010, web, 01 June 2015.

including: inflicting pain immediately after birth that may result in psycho-emotional damage; injecting 20,000 times the necessary amount of vitamin K into the single shot dosage given to newborns; and causing potential for infection with an injection when a baby's immune system is immature and birth naturally presents a host of bacteria, etc. to the new baby. Interestingly, Jewish boys were not to be circumcised until the eighth day of life (Gen. 17:12), which is argued the "only time in a baby's life when his prothrombin level will naturally exceed 100 percent of normal." As with vaccinations, vitamin K injections are given for convenience and profit, rather than according to the delicate balance of a human being. An obvious point made by Kate Tietje (Alternative Momma blogger) is that if all babies are given the vitamin K shot because all babies have deficient levels of vitamin K, then the lower level is normal. Holistic health is about working with nature rather than working against it.

Vaccines and the vitamin K shot can cause allergy because peanut oil is used in their formulations[131], which doesn't need to be listed as an ingredient since it is GRAS (Generally Recognized As Safe)[132] by the FDA. If the oil isn't processed perfectly, proteins remain. When proteins are injected and bypass the digestive system, they wreak havoc on the immune system and often trigger autoimmunity such as allergies. Some antibiotics are also cultured on peanuts. With the manner of immediately administering the vitamin K shot, vaccinating infants, and giving antibiotics to young children, it is little wonder why many have peanut allergies today.

My son has severe allergies to peanut, shellfish, and sugar-snap pea. During a time when a number of things compromised our son's health, vaccination harmed him. As is typical with one's first child, I labored longer with our son. After a day and a half, the doctor broke my water, nurses gave me Pitocin to induce labor (which had naturally started and stopped). I had an epidural and delivered our son without further complications. I was a nervous, overwhelmed new mother and stopped nursing after five weeks for fear that I didn't produce as much breast-milk as my friends, who were also new breastfeeding mothers. I introduced formula. Our son was very fussy and the formula did not seem to agree with him. At this time, the pediatrician vaccinated our son at his two-month appointment. I wish that the pediatrician had not injected our child with six vaccines at this acutely vulnerable time: DTaP (diphtheria, tetanus, and acellular pertussis), Hib (haemophilus influenzae type B), IPV (inactivated poliovirus), PCV and PPSV (pneumococcal conjugate), and Rota (rotavirus).

Thankfully, our son grew well and developed normally. As a small boy until he was about eight, he coughed until he vomited and suffered with asthma October through January. We gave him an albuterol inhaler, as his allergist advised, and a flu shot. The

131 "GRAS Substances (SCOGS) Database,"
http://www.fda.gov/food/ingredientspackaginglabeling/GRAS/SCOGS/ucm2006852.htm, FDA, 18 Mar. 2015, web, 01 Sept. 2015.
132 "Generally Recognized as Safe (GRAS)," http://www.fda.gov./food/ingredientspackaginglabeling/GRAS/, FDA, 04 June 2015, web, 01 Sept. 2015.

inhaler and the flu shot did not promote his health, and at this time, my husband began to apply more "old school" remedies to our son's body. After hot baths to open his lungs, my husband filled our son's socks with dried mustard before bed. He warmed milk with honey and butter to soothe the rattling cough. I was skeptical of these natural approaches and so were my family and friends. It didn't matter to my husband who is possibly the most stubborn person I know. God bless him. Along with the natural efforts to make our boy well, our son's body grew stronger as he began to play hockey. These years later, it is amazing to realize how our son's body has been strengthened by age, a more natural approach to health care and intense exercise on the ice.

We had a second son two years later. I breastfed through the first year, we had him vaccinated, and when he tried peanut butter on the tip of my shaking finger after he was two, he loved it. Five years later, my husband had decided we would not vaccinate our first daughter. Therefore, when she was born, I signed a release form and had the hospital pediatrician give her the standard hepatitis B vaccine when my husband went home for a shower. I had not bought into the notion that vaccines were unnecessary, or that they were harmful, until we met with Dr. Tenpenny when our daughter was a few months old. Thankfully, I had delayed scheduling the routine pediatrician visit at two months for her shots.

From our meeting with Dr. Tenpenny, my husband and I began researching as much as possible. We learned about the history of disease and sanitation as well as the prevalence of diseases in our country. It struck me as horrific and unexplainable when CBS News stated that the U.S. was first among industrialized countries for first-day infant mortality, with 50 % more infant deaths than other industrialized countries. I couldn't understand how 80 % of children with whooping cough had been vaccinated for pertussis. Pediatricians claimed that we just didn't know what whooping cough looked like, that society had been protected through herd immunity from this terrible disease. They never mentioned that those who had been vaccinated could still get the disease, but the information is available in multiple sources when a person is truly interested in comparing disease rates among those who have and those who have not been vaccinated. There seemed blind faith in vaccinations, despite the risks that were becoming abundantly clear.

I was interested in building natural immunity in the body with a balanced diet, clean water, and vitamins and minerals. Harmful chemicals seemed unavoidable and ever-present in the environment. At first, despite my growing distrust of vaccines, I was terrified that I couldn't possibly make everyone well enough to be safe against diseases without vaccines. This common way of thinking is absolutely incorrect when one realizes that vaccinations do not help us maintain a healthy immune system by injecting toxic substances into our bodies. In time, I realized that not vaccinating my children would allow them to be healthier. In the beginning of my epiphany, it had seemed an ironic and strange change of mind.

The shots themselves make us feel as though we're good, and now we won't get the measles. This is false confidence because individuals uniquely respond to this combination vaccine (currently administered with the mumps and rubella vaccine, MMR). This combination vaccine contains fetal stem cells and hen and rabbit eggs.[133] Despite an Internet search on Google that provides links sponsored by the government and institutions of higher learning arguing that vaccines do not cause autism, many stories from parents and studies that are published non-mainstream media argue otherwise. I do not discredit this information because it aligns with what I see. Unfortunately, believing that the vaccines do harm unsettles one's blind confidence in health care.

There are problems that the experts are not addressing. Details that explain why our kids are increasingly autistic are not accepted, and this is only one illustration: "Dr. Theresa Deisher, a PhD in Molecular and Cellular Physiology from Stanford University, and the first person to discover adult cardiac derived stem cells, determined that residual human fetal DNA fragments in vaccines may be one of the causes of autism in children through vaccination."[134] If doctors are not realizing potentials for harm, I had better, if I will to protect my children. It began to sink in to me that even if my kids ate cotton candy every night for dinner and didn't drink organic milk, I would help them to be well by opting not to vaccinate. I would aim to build their bodies strong with simple measures like active lifestyles with walks and play at the park, fewer fragrances and harsh cleaners, and eating organic apples, because these are available at Aldi's. My children eat the candy they get from school and the ice cream that loving Grammy enjoys with them. Life is short, and it is precious. Life is sacred, and I am grateful for those whom God has given to my care.

As I journeyed towards understanding vaccination, I was concerned with the prospect of my daughter encountering future contact with disease (because I hadn't known then that artificial immunity is short-lived and not lifelong). After all, many immigrants come to our country without having been vaccinated. Then I wondered why other countries don't vaccinate as much as we do in America. In 2011, Dr. Mercola argued that countries with the most vaccines have the worst infant death rate.[135] He reported that in the U.S. infants receive 26 vaccines, the most in the world. Yet, there is a higher infant mortality rate in the U.S. than in European countries. In 1,000 live births, six infants die in the U.S. In contrast, in Sweden and Japan, infants receive 12 vaccines, and per 1,000 live births, only three die. Additionally, the increase in sudden infant death

133 "Vaccine Overview," https://cogforlife.org/wp-content/uploads/vaccineListOrigFormat.pdf, Children of God for Life, 2015, web, 01 Oct. 2015.
134 "Stanford Scientist Proving DNA Fragments in Vaccines Cause Autism," http://edgytruth.com/2015/04/01/stanford-scientist-proving-dna-fragments-in-vaccines-cause-autism-great-read/. Edgy Truth, 01 April 2015, web, 01 July 2015.
135 Mercola, Dr. Joseph, "Studies show that the countries with the most vaccines have the worst infant death rate," Health Impact News, http://healthimpactnews.com/2011/studies-show-that-the-countries-with-the-most-vaccines-have-the-worst-infant-death-rate/, 2011, web, 12 Oct. 2015.

syndrome (SIDS) is arguably vaccine-related. Research illustrates that countries with the most vaccines have the worst infant death rate. In a study on "International Comparisons of Infant Mortality" reported by the United States Department of Health and Human Services in 2014[136], the U.S. had higher infant mortality than European countries:

> In 2010, the U.S. infant mortality rate was 6.1 infant deaths per 1,000 live births, and the United States ranked 26th in infant mortality among Organization for Economic Co-operation and Development countries. After excluding births at less than 24 weeks of gestation to ensure international comparability, the U.S. infant mortality rate was 4.2, still higher than for most European countries and about twice the rates for Finland, Sweden, and Denmark. U.S. infant mortality rates for very preterm infants (24–31 weeks of gestation) compared favorably with most European rates. However, the U.S. mortality rate for infants at 32–36 weeks was second highest, and the rate for infants at 37 weeks of gestation or more was highest, among the countries studied. About 39% of the United States' higher infant mortality rate when compared with that of Sweden was due to a higher percentage of preterm births, while 47% was due to a higher infant mortality rate at 37 weeks of gestation or more. If the United States could reduce these two factors to Sweden's levels, the U.S. infant mortality rate would fall by 43%, with nearly 7,300 infant deaths averted annually.

Dr. Richard Moskowitz argues that vaccinating entire populations results in more disease. He claims disease occurs in populations where people have been vaccinated, and vaccinating entire populations makes people less capable of fighting disease, which results in the development of different diseases:

> [V]accines can cause cancer and other chronic diseases. Prof. Robert Simpson of Rutgers raised precisely that possibility, in a 1976 seminar for science writers sponsored by the American Cancer Society: 'Immunization programs against flu, measles, mumps, polio, and so forth, may actually be seeding humans with RNA to form latent proviruses in cells throughout the body. These could be molecules in search of diseases: when activated under proper conditions, they could cause a variety of diseases, including rheumatoid arthritis, multiple sclerosis, systemic lupus erythematosus, Parkinson's disease, and perhaps cancer (55). Unfortunately, this is just the sort of warning that few people are ready, willing, or able to hear, least of all the American Cancer Society or the

---

136 MacDorman, Marian, et al., "International Comparisons of Infant Mortality and Related Factors: United States and Europe, 2010," http://www.cdc.gov/nchs/data/nvsr63/nvsr63_05.pdf, U.S. Department of Health and Human Services, 24 Sept. 2014, web, 01 July 2015.

American Academy of Pediatrics.[137]

With a growing resolve not to vaccinate our daughter, we began a quest for a pediatrician who would accept our decision. When I questioned a pediatrician about the need for our newborn to receive a hepatitis-B vaccine, he looked at us and said what we'd heard from three other doctors, what about the future, what if our child were ever in contact with the disease? At this point, I had learned that vaccine immunity was not life-long, which was the reason for booster shots. I distrusted the doctor who was either unaware of the limitations of vaccines, or simply trying to enforce a program that he had bought into. We were also aware that there were different types of vaccines: live, attenuated; inactivated, killed; toxoid, inactivated toxin; and subunit, conjugate. There was risk of shedding to others and even contracting the viruses after injection when the vaccine contained "attenuated" or live viruses in a weakened form, such as the measles, mumps, and rubella combination vaccine.[138] Dr. Tenpenny mentioned that illnesses could occur after vaccination with symptoms ironically like the diseases themselves. The doctor with whom we met didn't think this information relevant to our concerns with vaccination. My husband was stone still and rock-hard, his stubborn way speaking through his body, and the pediatrician seemed frantic, clearly agitated with my apparently calm husband. I knew this would not remain our daughter's pediatrician.

I had many questions about keeping our family well without vaccines (and without a doctor at this point). I thought of my mother's friend who had nine children and 12 grandchildren, none of whom are vaccinated. They are a very healthy family. In these 21 lives, none has autism, food allergies, or attention and developmental disorders. When the children are ill, the first choice of remedy is a cupboard of herbs and natural balms for normal childhood conditions. None of these children had diseases such as polio or hepatitis. When her active son stepped on a rusty nail, she cleaned the wound immediately with iodine, and then she soaked it in Epsom salts, and applied hydrogen peroxide. Her son did not get tetanus. Naturopathic doctor Dave Mihalovic argues that vaccination does not prevent the tetanus bacteria from harming the body because of the injection itself and because the vaccine does not produce lasting or effective immunity, as is evidenced from the boosters required.[139] Additionally, he explains, the bacteria are not a threat in America. Tetanus is not "communicable," and there can be no "herd immunity" from the vaccine. In fact, one cannot become immune from tetanus when

---

137 Moskowitz, Richard, "Richard Moskowitz, M.D. - The Case Against Immunizations," http://healthimpactnews.com/2015/richard-moskowitz-m-d-the-case-against-immunizations/, Health Impact News, 2015, web, 03 Aug. 2015.

138 Fisher, Barbara "The Emerging Risks of Live Virus & Virus Vectored Vaccines: Vaccine Strain Virus Virus Infection, Shedding & Transmission: A Referenced Report from the National Vaccine Information Center," http://www.nvic.org/CMSTemplates/NVIC/pdf/Live-Virus-Vaccines-and-Vaccine-Shedding.pdf, NVIC, 2014, web, 01 June 2015.

139 Mihalovic, Dave, "Why One Should Always Say No to the Tetanus Shot," http://www.vaccinationinformationnetwork.com/why-one-should-always-say-no-to-the-tetanus-shot/, Vaccination Information Network, 07 May 2013, web, 06 June 2015.

acquired naturally, or when vaccinated. And yet the vaccine and booster shots continue anyways. A booster shot is required every ten years, and the tetanus vaccine is typically administered with the vaccines for diphtheria and pertussis in children younger than seven (DTaP). In older children and young adults, Tdap is given: tetanus, diphtheria, and pertussis. Again, for adults, Td is a booster for tetanus and diphtheria. As Mihalovic explains[140], tetanus is ubiquitous—in and on the body, dust, and intestinal track of humans and animals. The problem is not the bacterium but the toxins that can produce under anaerobic conditions, only a threat when one lives in filth and is unwell to begin with. Even if tetanus were to develop, if a wound bleeds, there is no risk. If one is wounded and tetanus develops, simply draining the wound is the easy, effective answer. Most important is the health of the host, and no vaccine for tetanus (or anything else) can create stronger health. This is a fact: each vaccine necessarily includes animal and or human cells and harmful adjuvants. There is absolutely no safe and effective vaccine based on the necessary ingredients in each vaccine. Likewise, it is impossible to produce an ethical vaccine because of the very ingredients included in their formulation.

In addition to caring for her children with common sense hygiene, my mother's friend fed her family as well as possible (beginning with at least a year of breastfeeding), reduced chemicals in their home, and taught her children to do the same. When her children became sick with chickenpox and measles, they healed within a week, with little more than the nuisance of a cold. It was easy for her children to recover from illness because they had not had their immune systems over-taxed with antibiotics and various medications, including vaccines. Now her children have life-long immunity to diseases they simply recovered from. She continues very happy in her choice not to vaccinate her children, and her children agree, maintaining healthy immune systems of their 12 children without vaccines.

At the root of the vaccination problem is "organized denial" from scientists, academics, and health officials who refuse to admit causation between health problems such as autism and vaccination, even when the evidence is glaringly plain. Many medical professionals are trained to believe that vaccines are safe and effective. When a problem results, it isn't thought to be related to vaccination, even though, in many situations, doctors are unable to tell the patient why they are ill. It seems more important in current health care to diagnose the disease and to medicate the symptoms of conditions that may have been prevented.

Society needs doctors and scientists who are skilled and knowledgeable to acknowledge whole-person wellness, to teach a system of health care that denies it, and

---

140 Mihalovic, Dave, "Why You Never Need a Tetanus Vaccine, Regardless of Your Age or Location," http://preventdisease.com/news/13/050713_Why-You-Never-Need-A-Tetanus-Vaccine-Regardless-of-Your-Age-or-Location.shtml, 07 May 2013, web, 26 Jan. 2016.

to help patients build the body and feed the spirit. Physician Kelly Brogan[141] argues that health care providers and pharmaceutical companies, among others, work from an attitude of hubris, assuming that one can outsmart nature: "Humans suffer from *hubris* – we think we know better than nature, can fix it, manipulate it, and master it. There are (at least) two major transgressions that follow similar patterns, raise important red flags, and most certainly do not pass the sniff test: GMOs (genetically modified 'foods') and vaccination." She continues with the explanation of the problem that results from thinking that nature can be improved upon by science that is actually crippling us through GMOs and vaccines:

> Pharmaceutical companies and doctors think they can outsmart immune systems that have evolved to coexist with microbes, to be primed and educated by them. We are at war with infectious disease, and as a consequence, our fear and malice toward bacteria and viruses have lead us to compromise and alter our immune systems with pathogens entering our bodies through our muscles, accompanied by toxic additives that cripple our natural immune function and cause chronic inflammation.

It is human nature to act with a sense of pride, but we may instead listen to each other, learn, and be willing to change when experience and theory do not align. Rather than focusing on what another does not understand, aiming to imagine what she might could be an important key that very bright scientific minds could use to unlock the way in which whole theories of vaccination have failed us.

Most understand that wellness is complex and there is no easy answer, but even with this understanding, many good-intentioned doctors have faith in the current vaccine program. Some communicable diseases with low incidence of complication have been traded for life-long disorders. It is hard to understand why more medical doctors wouldn't realize the problem for what it is, but once we have been trained to think it is very difficult for each of us to change our minds, doctors included.[142] Some do because of scientific evidence as well as lived experience with human beings. Dr. Moskowitz claims:

> Nobody in his right mind would seriously entertain the idea that if we could somehow eliminate, one by one, measles, polio, and all the known diseases of mankind, we would be any the healthier for it, or those other quite possibly even more serious diseases would not arise and quickly take their place. Still less would a rational being suppose that the illnesses he or she suffered from were "entities" somehow separable from the patients who suffer them, and

141 Brogan, Kelly M.D., "Connecting the Dots: GMOs and Vaccines," http://www.greenmedinfo.com/blog/connecting-dots-gmos-and-vaccines, GreenMedInfo, 13 Nov. 2013, web, 06 June 2015.
142 Groopman, Jerome, *How Doctors Think*, Houghton Mifflin Harcourt, 2008.

that with the appropriate chemical or surgical sacrament such a removal can literally be carried out. Yet these are precisely the miracles we are taught to believe in, and the idolatries to which we aspire, forgetting the older and simpler truths that the liability to disease is deeply rooted in our biological nature, and that the phenomena of illness are the expression of our own life energy, trying to overcome whatever it is trying to overcome, trying, in short, to heal itself.

It is time for practices in health care to promote healing, and for each of us, patients and providers alike, to revere the sanctity of life. Working with nature, instead of against nature is at the heart of true healing. Diet, lifestyle, and holistic approaches that recognize personhood is body and spirit realign approaches to health care. Importantly, doctors and scientists who open the mind to what is possible by watching human beings naturally heal, would save so many of us from illness and death that comes as a result of theories that counteract nature. Consider the amazing cancer therapies (such as Coley's Toxins[143] combined with Gerson Therapy, and other immuno-stimulating and detox protocols) that are unheard of against the loud voice of chemotherapy and radiation, preferred today. However, as people reach out into alternative medicine circles, such healing practices may well revolutionize our society. Like all parents, we want our children protected for life from disease, and we do not want them harmed for life, or later in life, for the sake of short-term, artificial immunity. Parents (I suppose some would call "activists") and medical doctors continue telling of the harm that comes in the form of pharmaceuticals. We might listen, reconsider, try more natural ways to obtain and maintain wellness.

For example, activist and mother Jody McGillivray (who has a child with autism) argues for additional large-scale studies on the neurological and biological impact of vaccines and a large-scale study of the cumulative effects of the adjuvants in the vaccines. In a petition she composed to Representative John Boehner and Senator Harry Reid, she argues to repeal the Childhood Vaccine Injury Act of 1986, which would shift focus from production and mass distribution of vaccines to safe and effective vaccines as pharmaceutical companies would lose their immunity from claims of vaccine injuries.[144]

Medical doctor, Robert Rowen[145] argues vaccines cause harm because they include aluminum and injecting aluminum, and other harmful toxins into the blood, results in heavy metal toxicity. The body can handle a degree of heavy metals, as they are

---

143 CHIPSA, "Coley's Toxins: The History of the World's Most Powerful Cancer Treatment," http://chipsahospital.org/coleys-toxins-the-history-of-the-worlds-most-powerful-cancer-treatment/, Advanced Immunological Treatment and Research Medical Center, 2015-2016, web, 04 Feb. 2016.
144 McGillivray, Jody, "Repeal: The National Childhood Vaccine Injury Act of 1986," https://www.change.org/p/rep-john-boehner-repeal-the-national-childhood-vaccine-injury-act-of-1986#petition-letter, Change.org, 2013, web, 01 Sept. 2015.
145 When 1 + 1 = 100. A MUST READ PRIMER ON TOXINS Dr. Robert Rowen, FB, 3.18.15

"ubiquitous in the environment and we cannot help but ingest [them]," but repeated exposure injected into the body can "disrupt iron metabolism in cells, leading to injury." Rowan further argues for research on the synergism of components in vaccines:

> [I]t is rare, if ever, that the research looks into the synergism or explosive effects of combinations of additives or even "active" compounds. [...] here we are injecting toxins into infants when the infants already have some 200 known poisonous chemicals in their umbilical cord blood. We know that some of these chemicals, at the same levels are disrupting hormones in aquatic life and altering sex characteristics. And, we also know that there are areas of the country where toxins are in far greater concentration than others. It is this logic that compels me to discard (or look at them with a 'jaundiced' eye) studies and anecdotal observations, that vaccines do not cause injury. They simply have to. And the government and Supreme Court, and vaccine damage claims confirm this. But what we lack is knowledge of the toxic burden in any single child, and how his particular system may react to toxics, or, in the case of a lucky child with good elimination pathways, how resistant he might be.

Rowen continues with his argument on toxins and their synergistic effects on the body, particularly when injected and when the ingredients enter into the bloodstream, rather than when ingested by the normal entryway of the mouth or nose:

> The pundits of 'scientific' medicine give you descriptive names for the diseases they invent out of thin air, like 'social anxiety disorder.' But perhaps the real cause of the dysfunction is the toxins and synergism of a multitude of low concentration chemicals in our bodies. I'll close with this example. The FDA will tell you that the amount of Al in vaccines is 'safe.' And, it will tell you that the pesticide residue on your food is 'safe.' So for example, suppose 1 ppb (part per billion) of particular a toxin is safe. I can (very) reluctantly accept that for the sake of argument. (Actually, there is NO safe level of mercury or lead). But what happens when you combine 1 million different human made chemicals and toxins at 1ppb each? Now you have 1 million parts per billion of different mixed toxins. And the toxicity might be greatly potentiated by injection over ingestion. Indeed, even water itself is highly toxic if injected. It will poison your kidneys! It will lyse (break apart) your blood cells! (If that's all you knew about it, you'd classify water as a poison. The former is not a reason not to drink it any more than ozone's irritating effect by inhalation is not a reason not to use it for healing). In light of the above mercury-lead study (where 1+1 = 100), I don't even want to think about it. But our sick children aren't just thinking about it. They are actually living the nightmare in differing proportions each! Please wake up America!

Medical doctor Richard Moskowitz[146] explains how vaccines trick the body and break what the immune system has evolved to prevent by giving the virus immediate access to major immune organs and tissues without a way of getting rid of it. The result is an increase in the antibodies present in the blood, which has been argued a sign of one being "immune" to disease. Dr. Moskowitz argues that because of the viral elements in one's blood, the immune system actually weakens for an indefinite period of time and cannot respond to a host of infections (including strands of the disease one was vaccinated against). In many individuals, infection can occur without producing disease, because of the strength of the immune system, but if the immune system is overwhelmed by fighting viruses in the blood, more infections can produce more diseases in a person. His bottom-line argument concerning the functioning of vaccines is that it is misleading and a lie "to claim that a vaccine renders us 'immune' to or protects us against an acute disease," because it drives the disease deeper into the interior and causes us to harbor it chronically, resulting in progressively weaker responses to it and less tendency to heal spontaneously.

Aside from personal immunity, we have been taught that vaccines produce herd immunity and protection for others who may be too weak to be vaccinated. Herd immunity is only possible in communities where individuals have not been vaccinated and developed natural, life-long immunity to disease. Those who are vaccinated for chickenpox, shingles, MMR, rotavirus, and smallpox shed the "live" viruses for which they have been vaccinated,[147] and one with autoimmune disease is at risk by those who have recently been vaccinated. An unvaccinated, healthy person does not pose a risk for one who has a weakened immune system such as those with cancer, HIV, and autoimmune diseases. Doctors even warn patients who are infirm against contact with those recently vaccinated because some vaccines cause shedding of the viruses after vaccination. This has been long known, though too few realize the harm of getting the disease from the actual vaccine. For example, the vaccine (which had been a live oral vaccine) caused every case of polio since 1979. As explained earlier, vaccination programs abroad bring outbreaks of polio to the States because of the different strains of vaccination, the shedding of the disease, and the negative changes to the immune system that occur in one's body through vaccination.

The media leads people to believe that vaccinations are the only way to protect against diseases, failing to tell how vaccination harms many. For example, this past January (2015) a measles outbreak was reported in Disneyland. The risk of disease was delivered as though a horrific and new phenomenon. Dr. Janet Lebatin explains how the media created a "tempest in a teapot," meaning that this small event was exaggerated beyond its real importance. "The media, fueled by our government and the

146 Moskowitz, Richard, MD, "The Case Against Immunizations," http://healthimpactnews.com/2015/richard-moskowitz-m-d-the-case-against-immunizations/, Natural Impact News, 27 Feb., 2015, web, 01 June 2015.

147 "Vaccine Shedding," http://www.vaccineriskawareness.com/Vaccine-Shedding, Vaccine Risk Awareness, 2015, web, 05 Oct. 2015.

pharmaceutical companies, have taken what would ordinarily be a small unnoticed event and turned it into a media firestorm that is polarizing our country... for no good reason." She argues, along with others[148], measles is not such a serious disease. Most that are healthy and nourished heal and have lifelong immunity, and this creates true herd immunity, rather than false vaccine-induced herd immunity that wanes in most within five to ten years. She explains the history of the measles vaccine, which was introduced in the 1960s after the disease had been declining as a result of improved nutrition and healthcare. What's more, having measles, and other diseases, builds natural immunity: protection against some cancers, allergies, immunological, and degenerative conditions. She argues:

> When mothers were having natural measles during their own childhood years, they were passing much stronger and more protective antibodies to their infants during pregnancies and with breastfeeding. By the time maternally conferred immunity waned, the cycle repeated itself with natural childhood infections in their offspring. When widespread use of the vaccine became customary, we lost these protective biological dynamics.

The measles outbreak in Disneyland was relatively "very small when compared to other diseases and other causes of viral illnesses. There are many other causes of death and disability that the media has ignored, while stirring up a frenzy over measles." Dr. Lebatin states that in 2014 there were more than 600 cases of measles, and in the case that has caused all this hype there are 121 people affected.

It is frightening to see a bias so obvious in the media because it indicates that in our society, and nation, pharmaceutical companies monopolize wellness. There are simple and natural approaches that can help one maintain a healthy immune system. Dr. Lebatin concluded with ways to protect against diseases like the measles by supplementing with vitamins D and C, minerals, herbs, and homeopathy (the treatment of disease by minute doses of natural substances that in a healthy person would produce symptoms of disease).

In another example of the media misrepresenting cases of the measles as cause of national health concern, reporter Jeremy Hammond[149] addresses the story of a woman dying from the measles. The report came out in July, after the passing of a bill in California mandating vaccinations, but she had actually died in the spring. The last death

---

148 Bystrianyk, Roman, "Measles and measles vaccines: fourteen things to consider," http://www.vaccinationcouncil.org/2014/06/24/measles-and-measles-vaccines-fourteen-things-to-consider-by-roman-bystrianyk-co-author-dissolving-illusions-disease-vaccines-and-the-forgotten-history/, International Medical Council on Vaccination, 24 June 2014, web 01 Oct. 2015.
149 Hammond, Jeremy, "A Measles Death, Vaccines, and the Media's Failure to Inform: There is a Discussion to be had about Public Vaccine Policy. The Media Ought to have It," http://www.foreignpolicyjournal.com/2015/07/05/a-measles-death-vaccines-and-the-medias-failure-to-inform/, Foreign Policy Journal, 5 July 2015, web, 6 July 2015.

from measles was in 2003. The news went viral and prompted many to argue in favor of vaccines, especially in light of the "outbreak" in Disneyland in January. Hammond looks more closely at the situation, considering both sides of the "debate." The woman had additional complications and actually died of pneumonia. She had been on immune-suppressive drugs, and, in fact, Hammond argues that medical intervention caused her death. Most importantly, the woman had been vaccinated and had a "protective antibody titer" of the measles vaccine. She was a carrier of the measles and passed the disease to four others. It was through recombinant vaccine shedding that disease occurred, and this happens often. People argue that one who is not vaccinated is a risk to society, but in reality, when vaccinated with a live virus, a person sheds the disease for up to a month.

Hammond explains that vaccinating society creates temporary artificial immunity, which is less beneficial than cell-mediated, life-long immunity, and as a result, immune systems are naturally less able to fight diseases. Hammond argues that vaccines are automatically paired with herd immunity, though herd immunity is only possible in natural immunity, not through the antibody response that is theorized to protect the vaccinated. For the occurrence of herd immunity, society is exposed to disease and there is a low rate of mortality, which means that many had contact with the disease, survived, and are immune.

Herd immunity is predicated on the fact that living in symbiosis with viruses is actually good for the immune system, and, if one gets a disease and naturally fights it, one acquires lifelong immunity to the disease. Having had the illness actually "prime[s] the immune system of children to protect against other diseases." Vaccines destroy natural herd immunity and disrupt nature. Hammond explains that before 1963 doctors understood that the population would adapt and live in symbiosis with viruses. Since vaccines favor antibody response, vaccines suppress cell-mediated immunity. For example, when given the flu shot, the body does not produce natural cell-mediated immunity that would protect against more strains of the flu. Instead, one of the 200 strains is vaccinated against, and the risk of catching other strains with a less strong immune system is higher. Hammond argues that current research suggests that antibodies may not even be needed for development of immunity. Even with the measles vaccine, five percent do not develop a protective antibody, though everyone is advised to receive a booster shot. With a booster, three percent continue to be without the expected antibody response.

We no longer have natural herd immunity. This is why diseases are resurfacing. Esteemed medical doctors have been speaking out concerning the "myth of herd immunity," and yet it seems with the increase in vaccinations, their warnings are unheeded by pharmaceutical companies and the government. The pro-vaccine movement in current America frightens me for the future of our children and our children's spouses and their children. Life-threatening allergies and brain damage are very real concerns, indeed.

I was afraid when I began to change my mind about vaccines. It cost me trust and community to a certain extent. Convinced now that wellness is dynamic and particular to each human body and the balance it requires, anger is what I now feel watching current arguments on the mainstream media on "immunizing" our children. I hold forefront and center the most obvious point against vaccination: diseases were almost gone *before* vaccines were introduced. Diseases are eliminated by clean water and food and basic hygiene, like sewer systems, so that we do not have to live in filth. Today, we are oh so sanitized, and we are inundated with harmful chemicals and toxins that are sapping life. There is hope. We can choose to build natural immunity within the body with easy, clean eating and mildly active lifestyles. There is hope. We can choose to build the soul's immunity to despair through prayer to God, the Giver of Life, and begin to change ourselves and our small patch of the world for the good.

A trusted and wise friend mentioned that I would be going against large elephants that are only growing. "Do what you must. Then you will have no regrets." The following book is because there was no choice after studying the evidence that seems not to have been clearly, freely given to me and many I care about. We deserve to be informed of exactly what we put into our bodies, especially when we inject substances into the bodies of our newborns. Children are innocent and vulnerable. God help us.

When a situation wakes me up and I feel desperate for the Truth, I cry out to the Lord. In faith, I try to get it right—to understand, to act accordingly. Since my decision three years earlier to develop and maintain healthy immune systems, our family has been more well. My journey to understand vaccines has led to a journey to understand current health care in America. On a personal level, it has also led to deeper appreciation of life itself. It seems to me that there is a lack of reverence for the sanctity of life that is a gift from God. We often unknowingly buy into a way of tending our bodies, and the bodies of others, as though there aren't souls at stake. We must take every care to realize the body and spirit of each one of us is created by God and sacred. Vaccine harm is a significant problem because it layers family life with additional stress. Today's young families are overwhelmed by so many things, and becoming more whole could lessen anxiety and increase time available to give more attention things outside of illness and chronic health problems.

Once the Church learns that there are indeed fetal stem cells used in the production of vaccines and that vaccination has harmed the well-being of individuals from the start because of the ingredients used (preservatives, adjuvants, stabilizers; cell culture materials, inactivating ingredients, and antibiotics), an official position must be made declaring it unethical to vaccinate. After all, the Church issued its definitive statement back in 2001: the Holy Synod cannot condone manipulation of embryonic cells in any form for research purposes, including lines developed from destroyed embryos. This is precisely what is unequivocally occurring with vaccines. Orthodox Christians are to question the meaning of life, which, at this point in time, means especially that we must question current medical practices in order to determine if we are honoring life by engaging them.[150]

Though Illness and death are the result of a fallen world, life in Christ is a matter of preserving the sanctity of life. Jesus Christ saves us, and through our efforts to honor life and increase good in this world, He saves our neighbor.

---

[150] "Vaccine Excipient & Media Summary: Excipients Included in U.S. Vaccines, by Vaccine," https://cdc.gov/vaccines/pubs/pinkbook/downloads/appendices/b/excipient-table-2.pdf , United States Centers for Disease Control and Prevention, 6 Jan. 2017, web 7 Feb. 2018.

CHAPTER 4
Being Well in the Ancient Faith

I come to You, O Christ, blind from birth in my spiritual eyes, and call to You in repentance: 'You are the most radiant Light of those in darkness'.[151]

The body calls to the soul. When my period is late and I may be pregnant, the feelings and thoughts that follow my body's state alert me to what is in my soul. Emotions begin: fear, doubt—a touch of faith and hope; a rush of vanity, pride—and then a test. My body bleeds. Life is risked. All is on the line for an interim where I seem able to step nearly out of time. Eyes closed before a small "family protectors" icon in my kitchen as water boils. Tears loose against hot cheeks. The body is communicating to the soul, it is teaching humility, knocking against pride. My witness to others, visible from my actions, follows the deep and tender alone moments spent before my small icon in a space of time when it is clear to me that the Giver of Life is God alone. It seems that I only understand God as Lord when I let go of myself and trust in Him with my life. In my flesh and blood. In the deep recesses of my heart are those whom I love, and they are a part of my very being. I love God when my heart accepts His will be done: with me, with mine. In the moment of loving God, the past is absorbed and the future is, and goodness prevails without fear. I will for Life, for God Himself. "Your will be done on earth as it is in heaven...."

In the chapters that follow, I turn from the issue of vaccination to life becoming prayer. The topics are united in the notion that becoming whole is becoming more well in body and spirit. The Church is called a hospital. To me, when scripture says that Christians are to be in the world but not of the world, this is a call for Christ's healing presence in one's life to shine Light in the world. This light develops by one's life becoming whole in the Lord, and at the heart of this process is a Christian's approach to wellness as wholeness and holiness. The body and spirit are in constant relationship. Illness today is pervasive, and it is not merely a matter of physical ailments. Our souls need more attention through prayer in the name of the Father, Son, and Holy Spirit. When life is becoming prayer, everything done in the body should in some way complement life.

Prayer occurs on two levels: words that we learn to say and mean, and actions that follow from our hearts' embrace of God. Lives of the Saints recognized in the Church illustrate the power and transformation of the world through hearts and minds opening to God. The Saints' lives become prayers, and continue to change this world for the

---

151 Kontakion of the blind man, 6th Sunday of Pascha.

better through our remembrances of them. Unlike the Saints, in an effort to reintegrate personhood, we often turn to secular things instead of prayer, which can fill us only so much. Without prayer and personal relationship with the Father, Son, and Holy Spirit, we cannot be satisfied. According to George Morelli, our personhood is reintegrated by spiritual effort in the body:

> Integrating spirituality and personality takes intelligence, reason, and prayer. St. Paul told the Corinthians: 'I will pray with the spirit and I will pray with the mind also; I will sing with the spirit and I will sing with the mind also.' St. Maximus the Confessor taught that, 'A pure mind sees things correctly [and] a trained intelligence puts them in order.' A foundational building block of a trained intelligence is 'openness of heart.'[152]

The Saints, such as Elder Paisios, embraced this truth. The elder was canonized a Saint in the Orthodox Church in 1994 by the Holy and Sacred Synod of the Ecumenical Patriarchate of Constantinople on January 13, 2015. He was known for his gentle manner and acceptance of others. As a monk, he was conscientious to complete his obedience's and work among others, as well as maintain silence, in order to "progress in the art of prayer."[153] He thought that his own spiritual failures and lack of love were the cause of others' shortcomings. His sensitive nature pushed him to further his ascetic efforts of self-denial and pray for his soul and the world. He sought to understand peoples' reasons for events, rather than judging others. "The self-abandon with which he served God and his fellow man, his strictness with himself, the austerity of his regime, and his sensitive nature made him increasingly prone to sickness." Elder Paisios suffered respiratory problems for which he had to have a portion of his lung removed and blood infused by nuns who donated their blood for him. Additionally, he had a large hernia that was very painful and taxing on his physical well-being. His response to such suffering is an encouragement to each of us who suffers as "he bore his suffering with much grace, confident that, as God knows what is best for us, it could not be otherwise. He would say that God is greatly touched when someone who is in great suffering does not complain, but rather uses his energy to pray for others."

Eleutherios Tamiolakis[154] tells how he stopped worrying about the future after a visit with the Elder Paisios on Mount Athos. When the pilgrim arrived, he was greeted with, "I have been waiting for you," though the visit had not been announced. The Elder prepared tea and uttered "Glory to You, O God" as the impatient pilgrim grew more agitated by his patience and ease. Finally, the Elder asked why his visitor was so uneasy and nervous, "God will help you," he said.

---

152 Morelli, George, *Healing – Volume 1: Orthodox Christianity and Scientific Psychology*, Eastern Christian Publications, 2006, p. 16.
153 "Saint Paisios of Mount Athos," http://en.m.wikipedia.org/wiki/Saint_Paisios_of_Mount_Athos, Wikipedia, Aug. 2015, web, 15 Oct. 2015.
154 Sanidopoulos, John, "How I Learned to Stop Worrying About the Future," *Mystagogy* (Weblog), 08 July 2015, web, 15 Oct. 2015.

"Well, Elder, God helps us once or twice. Is He then obligated to help us continuously?"

"Yes, God is obligated to help you." The pilgrim was struck with the Saint's conviction, and the visitor's nervousness left him. Calm and peace overcame him. He listened as the Elder said that just as the visitor cared and would continually help his own children, God loved each of His children and was obligated to help them—through all time. One has no need to worry about the future because whatever comes, God is present and will always help. It may not be as one expects, and illness may persist, troubles may continue, because struggles can awaken us to the goodness of the Lord, our Savior and God. Elder Paisios promised the pilgrim and each of us by this story, that to trust and obey God brings us peace.

When I feel loved by God, I love others. I am on my knees, wrapped in incense, and the icons of Saints through the ages surround me. When I am near to God, I am open to this life. I listen to the hymns of the Church through others' strong voices, and the presence of the Holy Spirit abides in me. When I am united to all others who love God invisibly and visibly present, I sense God's personality. I bow down and worship Him, in silence. I have wept. He is loving and good, and His invitation to simply come is tender and sweet. As nothing but a shell of who I may become, weak against the distraction of my beautiful children, empty of compassion I wish I had, I come. As I am. Hardly able to realize the night falling outside against the fullness of life around me, I am absorbed and accept: I Am.

Christians are in Christ, and their lives are supposed to bring love to others in this world. This is so not because Christians are by nature more inclined to loving others. It is a struggle. One morning, the sky was cold and pink, and I sensed the mercy of God as I ran towards my street to enter into the morning craze of readying children for school and piecing back together an undone home. God loves each creation completely: each person is as important to Him as the next. This, indeed, is what God is: Love, full, unending, eternal, and all encompassing. I barely love myself, my babies, and those around me who are lovable, let alone others who upset me for one reason or another. God works in a heart open to Him, and such healing love can do many good things through a person's honest efforts. Even when a person does not know God, acting in love enables good and comes from God. On the contrary, evil actions lead to death and darkness.

Before Christianity[155], the Graeco-Roman world was cruel and inhumane. The sick were despised. Abortion, infanticide, and poisoning were practiced. Rosie Beal-Preston says,

---

155 Beal-Preston, Rosie, "The Christian Contribution to Medicine," *Christian Medical Fellowship*, 2000, web, 01 Sept. 2015.

The doctor was often a sorcerer as well as being a healer and the power to heal equally conferred the power to kill. Among the pagans of the classical world, only the Hippocratic band of physicians had a different attitude to their fellow human beings. They swore oaths[156] to heal and not to harm and to carry out the duty of care to the sick. The Holy Synod's address to the Church in 2001 reminds Christians of a physician's vow to do no harm. This physician's promise is stated in the Hippocratic Oath, which is applicable to this day as much as it was historically.

The Hippocratic Oath

I swear by Apollo the physician, and Aesculapius the surgeon, likewise Hygeia and Panacea, and call all the gods and goddesses to witness, that I will observe and keep this underwritten oath, to the utmost of my power and judgment. I will reverence my master who taught me the art. Equally with my parents, will I allow him things necessary for his support, and will consider his sons as brothers. I will teach them my art without reward or agreement; and I will impart all my acquirement, instructions, and whatever I know, to my master's children, as to my own; and likewise to all my pupils, who shall bind and tie themselves by a professional oath, but to none else. With regard to healing the sick, I will devise and order for them the best diet, according to my judgment and means; and I will take care that they suffer no hurt or damage. Nor shall any man's entreaty prevail upon me to administer poison to anyone; neither will I counsel any man to do so. Moreover, I will give no sort of medicine to any pregnant woman, with a view to destroy the child. Further, I will comport myself and use my knowledge in a godly manner. I will not cut for the stone, but will commit that affair entirely to the surgeons.

Whatsoever house I may enter, my visit shall be for the convenience and advantage of the patient; and I will willingly refrain from doing any injury or wrong from falsehood, and (in an especial manner) from acts of an amorous nature, whatever may be the rank of those who it may be my duty to cure, whether mistress or servant, bond or free. Whatever, in the course of my practice, I may see or hear (even when not invited), whatever I may happen to obtain knowledge of, if it be not proper to repeat it, I will keep sacred and secret within my own breast. If I faithfully observe this oath, may I thrive and prosper in my fortune and profession, and live in the estimation of posterity; or on breach thereof, may the reverse be my fate!

There were hospital-like centers in Buddhist regions. The Greeks practiced a simple form of medicine, and there were temples where the sick could sleep and recover. It is

---

156 "The Hippocratic Oath according to James Copland (1 March 1825)," The Hippocratic Oath, The London Medical Repository 23 (135): 258, 22 September 2014, web, 01 Sept. 2015.

said that the Romans established military hospitals.

Christians had a radically different outlook on the sick, disabled, and dying, and their perspective-changed society's way of caring for the weak and ill.

> Christianity gives men and women a new perspective and allegiance; their lives are spent in joyful grateful service of the God who has redeemed them and given them new life. In many ways, Christianity and medicine are natural allies; medicine gives men and women unique opportunities to express their faith in daily practical caring for others, embodying the commands of Christ; 'whatever you did for one of the least of these brothers of mine, you did for me.'[157]

Saints from the beginning of Christian history cared for individuals with a whole-person approach to wellness.

> [Many Saints] were doctors, or otherwise involved in the medical profession. Saint Paul, in his epistle to the Colossians, refers to the holy Apostle and Evangelist Luke as the beloved physician (4:14). The Great-Martyr and Healer Panteleimon was likewise trained in medicine. He is perhaps the most renowned of that company of saints called 'unmercenaries.' These are saints who freely donated their services, often healing spiritual as well as physical maladies. The unmercenaries have their own service in the General Menaion. In icons, they are traditionally depicted holding a box or vial in one hand and a spoon in the other. In the company of unmercenaries, we find three pairs of brothers named Cosmas and Damian, two pairs named Cyrus and John—and the holy women doctors and sisters, Zenais and Philonilla.[158]

Doctors of the early Church sought to heal individuals' souls and bodies. The Holy Martyrs Cosmas and Damian were physicians and miracle workers who labored without earning money. They were born in Rome during the third century and grew up Christian. They demonstrated gifts of healing and practiced medicine from an early age on. Emperor Galerius ultimately asked them to renounce their Christian faith in order to live, but they persuaded the emperor to believe in God when they healed him of a serious illness using their medical knowledge in the name of Christ. Eventually, a jealous physician led them out on the pretext of gathering healing herbs. As they journeyed, he stoned them to death.

The Christian emperor, Constantine, granted the first Edict of Toleration in AD 311. After this, Christians were able to give public expression to their ethical convictions and

---

157 Beal-Preston, Rosie, "The Christian Contribution to Medicine," *Christian Medical Fellowship*, 2000, web, 01 Sept. 2015.
158 Bushunow, Peter, M.D., "The Orthodox Christian at the Doctor's," Nikodemos Orthodox Publication Society, 2006, web, 01 June 2015.

undertake social reform. Christians cared for widows and the infirm with provisions that led the last pagan ruler, Julian, 355 AD, to comment that if paganism were to continue, they would have to treat those in need as well as the Christians. St. Basil of Caesarea (369 AD) founded a 300-bed hospital, which was the first large-scale hospital for seriously ill and disabled people. At the time, there were those victimized by the plague and leprosy, and others who were poor and or traveling, and St. Basil's care moved individuals to wonder about the love of God through the care of Christians. Christians helped others as would Christ, and monastic hospitals were founded with this basic premise.

As political freedom increased, so did Christianity and the care of the sick and infirm. Rulers, even those who were not Christian, were influenced by goodwill. During the Dark Ages (476-1000), cathedrals were to include a school, monastery, and hospital. In the Middle Ages, monks began to profess medicine and care for the ill, but it was said to interfere with their duties and so laymen were trained in medicine. This began the secularization of medical care and training.

In the eighteenth century, Christian hospitals re-emerged to care for those with cholera and fever, which broke out in epidemics, while others fled for fear of infection. Though not all, many doctors were at this time also Christians. As Beal-Preston says concerning Christian doctors, "commitment to love and care for those weaker than themselves as Christ did, people of faith were at the forefront of advancing standards of clinical medicine and patient care." Such doctors were ethical and upheld personal integrity, truthfulness, and honesty.

The Gospel shares how Christ was dedicated to healing the ill, and early Church doctors shared the same healing ministry. Beal-Preston writes that early on, Christians realized the connection between health and hygiene, and aimed to help society become healthier through more sanitary living conditions in prison, inner cities, and when dying. Christians also focused on world health, sending missions throughout the world in attempts to love others as one's self and to make disciples of all nations. According to Beal-Preston, the earth is full of healing, and God enables people who are skilled to make "use of healing, medicines, therapeutic diet practices, even surgical operations have generally been understood throughout history in the Church as appropriate, fitting and desirable ways of cooperating with God in the healing of human illnesses."

Throughout Christian history, and of course still today, the field of Medicine provides healing and help for the endless ailments of the fallen human condition. People have acquired and or deepened personal faith in God through both illness and healing, and God alone knows what He wills one to experience in order that that human person may turn more to Him. At times when ill, I realize that God is slowing me, and I am drawn to Him. Illness is humbling, and God knows this is good for the soul.

Whether weak or strong in the body, remembering God is key to opening the heart and allowing His mercy to work there. I aspire to be well, not ill, as the desire for wellness is innate to being human, and I am able to reach out to others when I am physically and emotionally stronger. Since my baptism eleven years before, I have prayed for the healing of soul and body each Liturgy and crossed my womb with a seal of faith. I believed that God was at work in my life and left many details in His hands with a faith that all things would be what they were meant to be. There were seasons when the pain in my heart was the only prayer I had, when words were dry and thoughts muddled. The hardest times were when our boys were smaller and cultural tensions pressed upon our marriage. My body was light and my heart so heavy. Because we had conceived the boys with fertility specialists, I hadn't imagined that we would have more children, but with faith the size of a mustard seed, God reveals amazing things, if, in doing so, good can increase. I believe that having a family increases my faith and draws me deeper into prayer.

When I am praying, with my mind and heart and through good works in my life, God's will arises from the circumstances of life. In each situation, the true test is to develop relationship with God, which draws us into Love. Oftentimes, it can seem to me that things should occur in ways that I will, but God alone knows what I need to learn love for others and to learn that God Himself is loving and good. Even the worst of situations, when a person chooses God, are opportunities to realize that God is good.

Being in prayer is not always something one realizes on a conscious level. The Holy Spirit, abiding in one who is in prayer, teaches us to love others, one's self, and God. The demons don't want us to pray, to make effort to love. Prayer leads to authentic relationship with God and to truly loving one another. Prayer is the difference between being a Christian and striving merely to be a "good" person. For anyone can change for the betterment of one's self, but change that occurs on the internal level of the soul transforms one's life and relationships with others. A Christian's faith grows with the experience of such transformational love.

In time, the depth of distance between my husband and me passed, and things began to appear differently, yet as through a haze. In a matrix of pain and resolve, I found hope in God, and the Mother of God helped and protected us in this time. When my husband's embrace was weak, a strength burned inside of me. I held him with confidence and amazing joy. Joy that sometimes wept but was refined and so true that it surprised me. It was a feeling, but then it was an action: a refusal to leave our cuddle on the couch, a rooted body beside the door, waiting for his return from work with fried potatoes on the stove. Something inside of me had been emboldened, it was joy that is known by fearless love, willing to endure pain and suffering for the beloved. Miraculously, even sorrow fed spiritual joy, and this gift of true joy came independent of life's situations. In deep dark patches, a light was powerfully visible to me, and it was strong and overwhelmingly good when I gave myself to it.

Love is a choice. Faith is renewed by staying when situations don't seem fair, by saying sorry and meaning it, by hoping that the other is better than limited vision allows me to understand in the moment. Faith increased as love grew and changed me, and by extension, my beloved began to feel my love warmer and more true. Once, I was walking back to our mini-van from class at the university. It was dark and drizzle was cold on my arms. A sudden urge to run to my husband, to the boy I'd made my life one with, welled up in me. I ran down a hill, slipping and sliding in mud, and returned home to his calm embrace. Little things like this have saved us, and these details of life that have had saving grace have come from willing for Love, fighting through the despair (sometimes in simply enduring it), and then, out of the dark, a ray comes. Loving one's spouse may develop the most when love seems missing and one feels desperate for the other.

Four years earlier, the boys were six and four, and I had thought that we would not have additional children. At this time, an orthopedic surgeon determined a rare yeast infecting my finger. While doctor's had ordered costly tests, it was a simple link to a yeast-free diet sent by my mother that helped me towards wellness. When I began to change my diet from high carbohydrates, veggies and fruits, to an increase in meat and dairy, my health improved. With the dietary change, my body began to feel better with much less stomach gurgling after meals and normal monthly menstruation cycles. I was astonished at these physical changes and thought of the many times I'd crossed myself in Liturgy and prayed for healing of soul and body. The healing of my body renewed my spirit. There was more I could give to my family. At this time, a subtle desire for another baby was growing within my heart. The Mother of God encouraged me as I prayed for her help, protection, and intercession to Christ for guidance concerning the changes I felt within me.

One evening, the mother of God was close at hand in the silent refuge of my bedroom. I held her icon to my lips, tears mingling into the aging wood, as the passing of time was palpably bittersweet. I wanted the children to grow and our family to mature, and yet I felt a loss for the uncontrollable ticking of time that spiraled life and its struggles into my past. It seemed I was not done giving of myself in a physical way, that I had just begun to understand love, and I wanted to give from this place of increasing faith. That evening, as I held the icon of the Mother of God, I thought about the Nativity. It was Christmastime. I could feel the light of anticipation present in our small home. I asked the Theotokos to pray to her Son and our God that my womb may be opened. The prayer came as breath, escaping my intentions that before had limited this prayer with conditions. As I asked her in that moment, I knew that we would have a baby girl, that she would be my gift.

It was a glorious time of Nativity, and a settling joy filled our home. My husband took time to be still. I laughed with the children and savored wrapping small gifts from Village Discount. Once, at Walmart, my older son and I passed a billboard with a baby girl. "I want a baby," I told him. He was surprised and told me he didn't think I would want another kid to make me crazy. We bought a small night-light with an image of a girl and the inscription: "Pray the Lord, my soul to keep."

During the day on the Eve of Theophany, I met with my mother and sister at Cracker Barrel for a light meal. I looked my sister in the eyes and told her that I would not be surprised if I had another baby. The day was crisp with light winter, and my mother and sister, and my nephew and son and I walked along a path after lunch. We laughed easily and gave piggyback rides to the boys. That evening, I took the boys to church with me and felt a glorious resurrection of joy burn within. Getting our coats on with Matushka,[159] I confided that I felt I might have a child.

A week later, it was an unseasonably warm pre-dawn in early January 2012. My sister was awake when I called her at four. The line on the second pregnancy test was clear and pink—it was not a "water-stain" mark, nor was the test's efficacy expired, as a nurse had cautioned me the morning before when the urine test at the doctor's office had been negative. Science proved what faith knew: I was with child. When I told my sister, she said that she hadn't prayed to the Mother of God or felt close to her before but she recently read a devotion about the Theotokos[160] being with the Christ Child and rushing happily to her cousin, Elizabeth. My sister expressed an understanding of the joy they shared in the holy conception of Christ, marveling at the miracle shared by these two women with deep love for one another and ever-increasing faith in God. "I know that Mary loves you so much, Lea, and that she's praying for you," she said. She confirmed the soft joy ablaze in my heart and I swallowed hard.

Our first daughter is the "gift" that my soul accepted her to be when I met with the Theotokos four years ago. The Lord is good and His mercy abounds forever. The demons do not want us to have relationship with God, to pray and experience personal encounters with the Theotokos and the Saints and with Christ Himself. When we do, realization of the Truth is transformational and never leaves us. Even when time passes, miracles are lasting impressions that God is true. The fear of the Lord engenders wisdom. To believe in God is to love those whom He entrusts us with, to preserve the sanctity of life. It is also to believe that He prepares us for what He has in store, down the road, for us to do and endure.

The wellness of my body encouraged faith and infused me with the desire to give more. A year after the birth of our daughter, my husband and I willed for another child. *If you both will.* She was also in God's plan. Half-way into the pregnancy, we were living with family and I was completing my dissertation. Stress mounted. As I tucked our daughter into bed for the night, I noticed the icon of St. Nicholas in the hallway. I peered into his eyes as though they really were windows to heaven and asked for help. There was calm as I drifted to sleep, and the burdens of life eased from me. That night, I had a nightmare that my eyes were being repeatedly stabbed, and I awoke shaking and afraid.

---

159 A title given to a priest's wife in the Russian tradition.
160 "God-bearer": the one who gives birth to God.

My husband had fallen asleep on the other side of the house on a couch, and in the dark room, I tremulously gripped the cross around my neck. As a sense of calm settled within me, there was a very fresh, slightly sweet aroma. I wondered what laundry detergent I had used, and sat up to peer through the dark at the end of the bed to see if clean clothes were there. Nothing was.

The next morning was stressful when I met with my dissertation advisor. I anticipated facing more of the same mental gymnastics that I had been enduring. As I sat in the office and was advised to again revise a number of details that would needlessly eat away time, the professor turned quietly to his computer. I glanced at the clock. I was supposed to be teaching but would not make it to class on time. I sat back and absorbed the silence in the room. The professor began to type on his computer. I prayed, "Lord Jesus Christ, Son of God, have mercy on me a sinner," in a spirit of calm acceptance. Trust began to replace control. As over a half-hour passed in quiet prayer, the fragrance from the night before returned. At first, I wondered what perfume I'd worn, but then it was obviously not a fragrance I owned but an otherworldly aroma that was so very pure and fresh. My face stung with emotion, and I believed with my heart that the Theotokos was near. After an hour, my professor turned back to me with the revisions he'd suggested, which he had typed out for me. I thanked him, and mentioned I would tell him something at another time. He asked me to please tell. In a mix of language that likely sounded very unclear to a man who prided himself on clear, logical argument, I shared that I had had a nightmare in which my eyes were stabbed, awoken to a beautiful fragrance that had calmed me entirely, and that this scent and feeling had returned here in his office. He said nothing, and I uttered goodbye. A feeling of Pascha filled my heart that day. The joy itself was enough proof that the aroma was from God.

As is often the case, miracles can fade and in retrospect seem like figments of one's imagination. Until something occurs that directly re-connects us to them. The Monday before our second daughter's baptism in the Orthodox Church, I placed her in her cradle, which was right below the icons in my room. She was content there and would stare and occasionally smile. An hour later, I went to check on her and picked her up. The fragrance I had experienced in pregnancy was on the top front of her hair. In doubt laced with faith, I prayed that if this were truly a divine gift it would remain for my sister and mom (who were visiting later that afternoon). I bathed the newborn with un-scented Dove soap, and the otherworldly sweetness remained, despite the cleaning. Once home from school, I asked my son to put his nose against his sister's hair, and he said that she smelled like church. Truth is often beyond words, given freely and embodied by the simplest among us, such as a babe.

Jesus Christ is the Master Physician, and faith in God makes us well in ways that modern medicine cannot. Throughout all ages, including current times, healing in the Christian Tradition pertains to the soul and body of mankind. When a person's life is becoming prayer, examining situations in life can change the mind and increase understanding. The older I get, the more I realize life is like a body of water. It pools in a place for a time, but is fluid and flows with the slight tilt of many forces out of my control.

The healing gift of love is spiritual food, it feeds the spirit, and it builds the entire body. Our family gathered at a pizza parlor to celebrate my parents' birthdays. The seven grandchildren bounced in the background with balloons and sugar-highs, bounding over to "Mimi" for birthday kisses. Early the next morning, my mother came over to watch my children. She had tears in her eyes as she thanked me for the celebration. She said that as she drove through the frozen February morning, the sky was so blue and her heart so full with joy in the Lord. My mother inspires me to appreciate the fleeting moments we share. Having a blast differs from the joyful peace she felt, and she understood the difference to be a gift from God.

Looking back on the past fifteen years, it's miraculous how my marriage has been good for my soul. By the grace of God, I am more well now than ever before. A decade earlier, I wouldn't have thought that my husband would serve as a catalyst for my wellness, but now I do. We are very different from each other, and to maintain a loving relationship we have had to listen to the other with patience and self-sacrifice, which we've often taken our time to acquire.

Loving is in ways like acquiring taste for particular foods. Before my husband, I had been a bread and butter, with a side of salad, kinda-girl. But my husband simply loves things salty, meaty, cheesy, and garlic-spicy, and his approach to eating is like his approach to living: he savors the flavors of life and is patient to get a meal just perfect. He's helping me balance food groups and appreciate good things in life. On date nights at home, my husband grills salmon and we chop salads with raw garlic and sip Moscow Mules (vodka and ginger beer with lemon slices). Our girls are usually weaving between our legs, pushing their loud toys, while the boys are lounging with an electronic, until Daddy gives an order to "set the table." Energy divides us between the baby in her highchair and the son who is complaining that our food is not normal food that he likes. I share about the Dormition Fast, and our eldest son asks about Mary. "What did she do?"

"She led a quiet life. She gave herself to God first, and she took care of His home." I drift into an imagination of what it may have been like. It makes me think of the beauty of a family unit, the closeness that can be there, and the simple time we have in a moment to realize that God is yet still with us.

It dawns on me that my husband and I have spent over half of our lives with each other. Though many things have been added: children and extended family, a home and jobs, it feels familiar with my husband in a way that it always has. There is Presence with us, Love. God felt near, even before we were baptized in the Orthodox Church, but there is a growing responsibility I feel to understand the Faith and to let the Truth of God change and save me. Each of us has a choice to accept God, to have faith in Him, to be willing to change. It seems to me that this is not a one-time choice to believe in God.

Rather, it is a lifetime of choices that establishes relationship with God, and this is what it means to pick up my Cross and follow Christ. It is anything but easy for my life to become prayer, but if my life becomes prayer, others around me sense peace that flows from the Holy Spirit at work in me.

Saints are created in all times and in all places by the challenges of a given life. It is not the ease but the demands of one's life, which become a refining fire. Some have left the world to travel through deserts in a one-on-one life with God. Some slept on rocks and barely slept at all; others ate bugs and lived in caves, deserts, or deep recesses of the forest. As the children turned upside down the living room, it could seem easier to be a monastic than a mother and wife.

It takes effort to be well, and it takes effort to be saved. It may seem easier to throw in the towel, to eat French toast and watch cartoons, rather than make the push for Divine Liturgy. It may seem like more fun for my children to play at home than to go, again, to church (Great Lent, in particular, has many services). But when the details are examined, it is better to go. In going to church, we enter an aroma of holiness: the church calls with a loud bell, incense rises in the crimson sanctuary, full of icons and the spirit of eternal life. Candles glow before the Mother of God as I pray with the baby in my arms, toddler at my heals, and son beside us—roaming his finger through the small candle flame. The struggle is real as I juggle books and baggies of cereal, repeat for the kids to be quiet, try to keep all together and steal moments of realization that God is here—that He is everywhere. But we have come, and it is better than French toast, because in coming to a place so full of life in Christ it begins to become easier to realize that God *is* everywhere present. When Holy Communion is taken, it fills me so perfectly, as though nothing else matters and all is right.

It was Annunciation, a feast during Great Lent in honor of the Mother of God's acceptance of Archangel Gabriel's news that she would provide the Christ child's humanity. Mary was a humble woman, without money or reputation. She was a girl raised in the Temple where her parents had taken her as a toddler in fulfillment of their own promise after finally conceiving a child late in life. Angles fed her. I wished the angles would feed my children, as we struggled to "saddle up" and get across town for Liturgy. The children and I arrived early, and the boys chased each other, their small sister laughing and following behind them. *Don't throw pinecones at each other; get outta the mud; either in or out of the van*—it seemed easier to go into the church's nursery with all of them. At least there we'd be contained and calm down before service. The eight-year-old soon found lint tape with which new games could arise, and I gave in. Borrowing my I-phone, the older boy video-recorded my introduction of the Povozhaev dramatization: "Blond Mr. Beans are known to be quite hairy. Some use tape to get rid of that problem." Brother then used the tape to clear his imaginary armpit hair. Sister pushed into the drama at the end by flat lining her brother to the ground and laughing.

We finished up in the nursery, inching towards the sanctuary. It was time to settle down and enter Liturgy. With a half-hearted sigh I thought, *Here I am, Lord, and the children You have given me.* I didn't feel well, and faith seemed transparent, flimsy. I moved us into the sanctuary because I believed in God. We came to service because it was the day to realize the Announcement to the Mother of our God, a day that occurs each year, and may be experienced uniquely each feast of Annunciation. I believed that sharing the Faith with my children on earth would provide a foundation for them to choose to follow God as they grew. Because I longed to share joy with them in the Kingdom of Heaven, we had come. It was so simple: a desire and a decision to go because it *would* be good. But it didn't yet feel good.

A sick man came late to the service as I paced with the baby in the back of the church. His raspy voice hymned the Creed, and I sang with him. There was a powerful feeling of life—chills crawled up my neck. I felt close with those around me, even though I didn't know anyone. We sang:

> My thoughts, like thieves, have seized me, a wretched man. My mind has been robbed, and I have been sorely beaten. My soul is wounded, and I am stripped of virtues. I lie naked in the highway of life. The priest saw my pain and hopeless wounds and looked away. The Levite could not bear my groaning and passed me by. But You were pleased to come, O Christ my God, not from Samaria but from the flesh of Mary. In Your love for mankind, grant me healing, and pour upon me Your great mercy![161]

Experiencing God—and the holistic wellness found only in Him—is the reason to go to church, and the reason to bring children to church. The next day, my mother and sister were over and we talked in my kitchen while our children chaotically played about us. "You would beckon us down from the cross, Mom! You'd weep for us to come enjoy some jellybeans!" We all laughed. Our mother didn't want us to suffer, and I could understand when I thought of my own children. But more than my hope against pain and suffering, I desire with all of my heart for my children to experience a living love for God that calls to them as they go through life and its many struggles and temptations.

God knows in 2015 America that there is pain and suffering, and the healing we desire is a deep-seated need. I can feel overwhelmed and depressed when I consider the future with government passing bills allowing prescription drugs with less testing of safety and long-term effects; with mandatory vaccinations; with Arizona's air-force base displaying gay pride flags in place of the United States of America flag; with the slaughtering of Christians throughout the world; with the U.S. government threatening to amend the Constitution so that we may not have the right to bear arms, even as the

---

161 Leavetaking of the Annunciation, triodion, tone 8.

government buys out ammunition, militarizes its police force, and readies camps for reasons unknown to the public.

It isn't surprising that America's youth are despondent. They do not know, have not been taught, right from wrong. Few have been pushed to focus, sacrifice, and work good. Parents have a responsibility to teach their children how to be well, body and soul, but parents today are often unsure, or value what isn't most essential. My mother said that God shows Himself to us. His mercy alone saves us from ourselves through visions of hope in Love. When the overwhelming sense of this world going to hell in a hand-bag weighs upon me, there is comfort in knowing that in all times and places God saves souls. It is possible to be well, and I cherish others who help me realize ways to become more well. God is saving this troubled, broken world, even still.

Tears are said to clean the soul. A very strong woman wept in her kitchen over her husband's recent decision to leave. She couldn't believe that over half of all marriages failed. That so many had to endure the tortures of divorce. It continued to astound her that her husband could choose to leave the family. In meeting with the priest who had married her and her husband, she was asked about feelings of anger and pride. She realized these feelings in her heart, but in her tender, soul-wrenching confession, she said that what hurt the most was that she feared she was responsible for her husband's spiritual fall. She loved him enough, despite his leaving, to break inside over his sin. She did not will for him to divide from her and that hurt, but she mourned even more over his choice to act in sin. Only in true love can one realize spiritual truth and weep so completely for another.

Family life today is hard, maybe it always was. Years ago, when there was intense stress in our family, my priest once told me that he liked having me at vespers, but it might be better to stay home and spend time with my husband. These years later, a friend encouraged me to attend vespers. It was after 4:00 p.m. Saturday evening when my husband and I finally crossed paths. The house was quiet as day transitioned to night. In silence, we sat on the carpet with the baby. My husband said that he would golf on the morning of Father's Day, instead of attending Liturgy. My heart plummeted. Another too-busy Sunday, another round of excuses. The cycle of frustration began in my heart, and I was ready to stand up and shower, to take myself out of the house and go to vespers.

I couldn't move from the carpet. Something about the peace of the softening light through the window, the quiet between us, the sober sense that love was not boxed into a place and a time. To love my husband was to let it go—his choice to golf and my hard-heart that could storm me off to vespers. The Church has vespers because it is good to attend prayer services and to maintain a cycle of praying, but our very lives are to become prayers and this sometimes means choosing to stay home and spend time with those God has allowed in my life.

The beauty of Holy Orthodoxy is in the manifold opportunities found within the Tradition that helps me change my perspective and better understand the meaning of love. In a prayer of St. Basil the Great in preparation for Holy Communion, the following words speak of the spiritual and physical reality of being a Christian: "[L]et Thy holy things be for my purification and healing, for enlightenment and protection, for the repulsion of every tempting thought and action of the devil which works spiritually in my fleshly members." I believe that God reveals Himself, as He wills, for the salvation of my soul, and that He often does so through my own body. Because I long to be saved, I pray. Because a relationship with God is saving me, I am changing. By the grace of the Holy Spirit, I am saved from the limitations of my understandings. As a result, I am becoming well.

CHAPTER 5
Life as Prayer: The Warring Dogs

Prayer is a permanent communication between man and God, whether one uses words, music, or silence. The Holy Fathers ascertain that to pray is the presence of God within us. One has to feel this presence as a pregnant woman feels the presence of the babe in her womb. Prayer is not a ready-made or a recited formula but it is a state of spirit. [....] Agony is also an indication that God is with us. Many times God inspires awe and sacred fear and trembling, not only sweet and comfortable feelings. Many times we have to cry out in despair. Being asked by the disciples, 'Lord, teach us to pray,' Jesus answered by giving them a text, not a method. There is no trick, no technical skill to prayer. Just pray, and the Holy Spirit will reveal your own way to you.[162]

All icons are images of Christ. Their faces are to be the Face of Jesus Christ. Christians alive on earth are as icons of Christ as well, when He is seen by the manner in which one lives his life. My priest said that mankind was created in the image and likeness of God before Jesus Christ came to earth and took on flesh. God has always been: the Alpha and Omega, without end, and all of life attests to Him. A human being is much more than an automaton because God is Love and created every person to uniquely express that boundless Love. With life comes the responsibility to choose God and so to exert effort to please God, or to settle and defend myself-as-I-am-is-good-enough. It is not easy to choose God in this fallen world, and there is a thin line between sinner and saint. Most of us are tottering upon a middle road that includes sin and effort made to receive God, be forgiven, and experience salvation. The process of facing Christ is continuous, and when His mercy and grace saves, living prayer, as a person's life, shows the world God Himself.

Unfortunately, knowing this in my head doesn't change the fact that I do not tend to live in a way that presents a sweet fragrance of Christ to others, let alone to God. My husband wore his tuxedo-printed t-shirt and khaki cut-offs, and looking at him sitting at the table with my sister and parents I saw a mix of the boy-man who's humor and youth was about to give way to man-talk. As the conversation grew heated and controversial, my voice was anything but respectful. My husband and I didn't hold back our frustrations at the other's dominance in a conversation with my family on religion and politics that could go nowhere fast. We were biting and disrespectful to one another, and we insulted my parents and sister in our disregard for their feelings and differences of opinions. My sister mentioned that we are the most passionate couple she knows. I think my husband found this a sort of compliment, but I was tear-struck and snapped at her. Thus began an

---

162 Braga, Fr. Roman, "The Method of Prayer," *Life Transfigured*, vol. 16, 1, summer 2015.

ugly, stinking illustration of myself-as-I-am-is-good-enough. Self-control was out the window. I left the house with my parents, sister, and our children for a walk in the late afternoon sunshine feeling unworthy of Peace, despite having partaken of the Eucharist earlier that day.

My family walked along the lake at the end of my street in silence. I felt raw. I wasn't ready to reach out to God, not yet. I was too full of my mind, too frustrated by my failures to be self-controlled and loving. I justified my feelings. It wasn't as if I were a nun; I had passion and opinions, and so what if I'm not perfect. I felt miserable. Annalisa Boyd quotes John Chrysostom on the opportunity to work for the good in each one's unique life:

> You greatly delude yourself and err, if you think that one thing is demanded from the layman and another from the monk; since the difference between them is in that whether one is married or not, while in everything else they have the same responsibilities.... Because all must rise to the same height; and what has turned the world upside down is that we think only the monk must live rigorously, while the rest are allowed to live a life of indolence.[163]

People, especially my loving family, knock against my "rough edges" far too often, thank God. Marriage in particular challenges me to understand and love. To build a loving marriage is a holy pursuit meant to create a peaceful home, and this endeavor is also necessary for my own salvation.

It's funny—perhaps tragic—how different men and women tend to be. In a blog post by Dave Willis[164], he discusses the importance of understanding a spouse's needs. He says that women need their husbands to help them feel loved, beautiful, held, communicated with, and thought of on a daily basis, and that men need their wives to help them feel respected, reflected upon, sexually satisfied, productive, and strong.

Living prayer is life in Jesus Christ. I think of this relationship in terms of the five needs of a husband and the five needs of a wife. Every day, I must show God my love for Him and express gratitude for the beauty of this life. Every day, I must hold my children and savor the gift of life, communicating to them my love and adoration through the perfect goodness of the Holy Spirit abiding in me, even though I am so far from perfect I am barely even decent sometimes. Nonetheless, if I will to simply love those in my every day, then the Holy Spirit is present for others through my life. Daily, my thoughtfulness provides a channel to God, no matter what hells on earth threaten me. Every day, God desires my respect, reflection on His presence in my life, and the intimacy of my obedience to Him. As a temple of the Holy Spirit, the words that come from my mouth,

---

163 Boyd, Annalisa, "The Ascetic Lives of Mothers," Ancient Faith Publishing, 2014, 18.
164 Willis, Dave, "Five Things Your Wife Needs Every Day," http://www.patheos.com/blogs/davewillis/5-things-your-wife-needs-every-day/, Patheos, 29 Mar. 2015.

like the activities of my feet and hands, should foster holiness in my heart. More times than not, though I rarely realize it, I'm like a fish flopping out of water in need of gentle help to get back in: Lord have mercy.

I was in the kitchen with my eight year old near bedtime. He was eating toast and viewing a YouTube video of his favorite video-game, Mine-craft, as I read. It was the fourth week of Great Lent, and a desire to pray a little bit more grew inside. When I prayed in the morning before the children awoke and before I had to teach at a local college, my mind sometimes drifted: thoughts of people, of things to do, of various worries crept up. At times, a hot, fast distraction stole peace. Despite my splintered mind, prayer was growing inside my heart, working there, and a hunger-like desire for God subtly increased. There was a sense of Presence, and because of this I longed to continue in prayer, but I also felt afraid. To pray, I had to face myself, and my shortcomings pained me. I was proud and vain. I was too self-conscious of how I appeared to others, even in church.

Walking up for Holy Communion, I barely grasped that it was Christ Whom I received. Archimandrite Sophrony writes, "The whole of our Christian life is based on knowledge of God, the First and Last, Whose Name is I AM. Our prayer must always be personal, face to Face."[165] I looked up from the article and at my son who was drawn fully into the laptop. I called to my boy: "Listen to me, come from this other world," I begged.

He asked me, "What mom?" How distant we could be, even though so close together. Like in step for Communion, how far from God, even with the occasion to be with Him. The heart is distracted, racing against itself. One may utter prayers; think of the Saints, think of God Himself, but this was not prayer. This was not talking with my son.

"I love you," I told my son. "Listen to me, please. I just realized that we can pray and fail to know God. We must seek Him and develop a personal relationship with Him." My son looked at me with an open face. "When I die, don't just remember me. Pray to the Lord for my soul. Talk to me, and talk to God for me." He said that he could see what I meant. God bless his tiny soul, my blonde, stubborn-like-mule, sweet one.

The next day was Sunday, and the sun was blindingly bright and hot. We commemorated the image of Christ "Not Made by Hands," and our priest spoke on the importance of face-to-face relationships. Even those who are blind may touch another's face to get a sense of the person with whom they wish to relate, he said. A person is known by the face, and this is even the case with Jesus Christ, as the story of this icon shows. According to the Tradition of the Faith, during the time Christ was on the earth,

165 Sophrony, Archimandrite, "The Jesus Prayer: Method," http://beforeitsnews.com/christian-news/2013/10/the-jesus-prayer-method-by-archimandrite-sophrony-2484080.html, Before It's News, 08 Oct. 2013, web, Mar., 2015.

teaching and healing, a ruler of the city Edessa in Syria, Abgar, had leprosy and wanted the Lord to come and heal him. The Lord replied to Abgar's messenger that He could not at that time go to help Abgar. Jesus Christ wiped His face on a towel and sent it with the messenger back to Abgar, promising to send an apostle to heal him. When Abgar received the napkin, upon it was an image of the face of Christ. In faith, Abgar praised God and began to heal. When Thaddeus later came to heal Abgar, he had already healed. The Apostle Thaddeus baptized Abgar and everyone else living in Edessa at this time. Abgar wrote on the Image Not-Made-By-Hands, "Christ-God, everyone trusting in Thee will not be put to shame," and adorned it over the city gates, as it was the first icon of Jesus Christ.

A friend recently had a beautiful baby girl with her new husband. She also has a daughter who is 21, and another daughter who is 12. My friend came from Russia when she was a very young women. Her parents divorced, and she had to find her way in America as a young, single mother. She married and had her second child, but her husband hadn't been interested in living for God. This was a time of struggle for my friend, whom I met at church when I was converting and dealing with my own transitioning family. My friend prayed for a husband, the right man who would be able to care for her and share faith in God. After years, she married a man that my husband had come to the States with in childhood, both he and my husband played hockey and were from the same city in Russia. My friend's new daughter was baptized "Maria," after St. Mary of Egypt. This Saint had been a prostitute through her youth. Her beauty had lured men to her during a pilgrimage to the Holy Cross. When she reached the church and was unable to enter the doors by an unseen, though sharply felt power, she realized her sinfulness. She repented deeply, her entire body and spirit longing for cleansing that would take her into the desert for the rest of her days. She fled, moving against her desire and physical pain, to mortify herself in repentance. The choice she made came in a moment, and was enough food to last the rest of her life. I wept when I first heard the baby's name. This little girl is an image of beauty that comes from faith, patience, and trust in God.

I have a photograph of an icon of St. Seraphim of Sarov. He is slumped over and leaning on a cane. For years, I didn't know who this icon depicted. Now that I do, he is thumbtacked beside my bed. St. Seraphim of Sarov's life was a humble, living prayer. He led a Christian life that inspires many still.[166] He was born on July 19, 1754 to pious parents and named Prochorus. In his childhood, his parents built a cathedral, but before its completion, his father died. His mother continued with their building project and lived a pious life as a widow. Once, his mother took him to the cathedral where Prochorus fell from the bell-tower seven stories high. Though he should have died then,

166 "Repose of the Venerable Seraphim the Wonderworker of Sarov – Orthodox Church in America," OCA, http://oca.org/saints/lives/2015/01/02/100008-repose-of-the-venerable-seraphim-the-wonderworker-of-sarov, 2015, web, 01 Oct. 2015.

the Lord preserved his life. Prochorus had other close calls with death as he grew. In childhood, he became ill and saw the Mother of God in a dream. She told him that he would be healed, and the following day a church progression came through his courtyard. He kissed the Kursk Root Icon of the Sign, and was healed. His mother knew of his desire to become a monk, and she blessed his path to righteousness early in his life. With her blessing, the young Prochorus served as a monastic in the Sarov wilderness monastery. There, by constant work, he guarded himself against despondency—a danger for new monastics, and for anyone changing with feelings of being alone. With prayer, silence, work, reading of scripture, and patience, a novice is protected against the demons of acedia (or sadness), who try to re-route a monastic's efforts to develop life as prayer.

Prochorus increased his efforts to know God, and the grace of the Holy Spirit was within him. His spirit and body developed a distinctly Christian humility that drew seekers to the Lord. He labored in the monastery for eight years and fasted from food Wednesdays and Fridays before he was tonsured a monk and named "Seraphim." The following year, he was ordained a hierodeacon. While serving, Seraphim saw angels with the priests.

A great miracle occurred in St. Seraphim's life on Holy Thursday. After the little entrance with the Gospel during Divine Liturgy, he lifted his hands with the prayer, "O Lord, save the God-fearing, and hear us, unto ages of ages." He looked up and was blinded by a bright light. He saw the Lord Jesus Christ coming through the western doors of the temple, surrounded by the bodiless powers of heaven. Christ walked to the raised platform in the nave of the church and blessed all those praying before entering into His icon to the right of the royal doors. St. Seraphim was unable to move or speak following this experience. He was led into the altar and stood another three hours in silence.

After this vision, Seraphim intensified his spiritual efforts. He toiled at the monastery during the day, and at night he prayed in his cell in the Sarov forest. In 1793, he was ordained to the priesthood. He served the Divine Liturgy every day and continued in his ascetic efforts. He became the new Superior of the monastery, and he devoted himself to solitary prayer. In a life increasingly becoming prayer, he ate once a day, memorized hymns and prayers, and continued in the Jesus Prayer. He often didn't see others nearby him because of his singular focus. He was in such a prayerful state working in a garden when robbers came upon him and beat him nearly to death. Again, he had a vision of the Mother of God and was healed. He spent three years in silence, separated from the world, and gained a peaceful soul with full joy in the Holy Spirit.

St. Seraphim led a Christian life marked by great humility. He focused on God and experienced love and peace. St. Seraphim's life was a mix of silence and interaction with others, and his activities were informed by the divine presence of God. Knowing the saving and healing love of God showed St. Seraphim the way to help others:

The Elder saw into the hearts of people, and as a spiritual physician, he healed their infirmities of soul and body through prayer and by his grace-filled words. Those coming to St Seraphim felt his great love and tenderness. No matter what time of the year it was, he would greet everyone with the words, 'Christ is Risen, my joy!' He especially loved children. Once, a young girl said to her friends, 'Father Seraphim only looks like an old man. He is really a child like us.'

St. Seraphim realized the awesome presence of God and didn't feel alone when he was in the wilderness. When he returned to the monastery after 15 years in the forest, he continued to live in solitude. At that time, the monks among whom he dwelt observed his ascetic life. In another vision towards the end of his life, the Mother of God told him to end his solitude and receive others. St. Seraphim obeyed God. He spent time with monks, nuns, and pilgrims and by his life showed the Holy Spirit. When asked how one could know the Holy Spirit is with us, St. Seraphim's eyes flashed like lightening and his face shone like the sun. The one looking upon him perceived the Holy Spirit.

St. Seraphim focused his mind and heart on prayer, and his body acted with self-control, strict fasting, and continual labor. Though a secret until after his falling asleep in the Lord, St. Seraphim was said to rise from the ground in prayer. At the end of his life, St. Seraphim said, "Save your souls. Do not be despondent, but watchful. Today crowns are being prepared for us."

Saints strive through ascetic effort against the vices: wrath, greed, sloth, pride, lust, envy, and gluttony. Through the Holy Spirit's presence in one's life, abiding in one's heart, a human being is saved. The Saints show how to make effort through good works and acquire virtues: chastity, temperance, charity, diligence, patience, kindness, and humility. God's presence grows inside of those whom He is saving. The gifts of the Holy Spirit: wisdom, understanding, counsel, fortitude, knowledge, piety, and fear of the Lord, testify to His Presence in one's life. A Christian aims to return to God's good intentions for her soul, which results in a joyful heart—though in the course of the struggle happiness cannot be felt at all times.

Despite all else, the mark of a Christian's life is joy. Joy is present because God is present. In obedience, one cooperates with Him, and the Kingdom of Heaven grows inside a person's heart. I often experience joy after Holy Communion that differs from happiness on other occasions. It is an otherworldly, exuberant feeling of release. Nothing matters so much as it had, as it will again. I believe in Christ because He is Living Joy in my heart. I do not feel this all of the time. Other times, I yell at the children to vent the pressure; I begrudge my neighbor whose bonfire has my son's nose to the window instead of the pillow; I hide goodies from my husband so there's chocolate leftover in the morning. Though I am far away from sainthood, even I can experience Christian joy that saves my soul because it keeps me hungry for God. To taste and see how good He is, I prepare myself before Liturgy, in whatever ways I can muster, so that my heart is open and able to receive His love. This lifetime is all about learning to love God and others.

This is the process of life becoming prayer, and it is how a person becomes Christ-like, which is infinitely deeper than mere affiliation with a religion.

One of my spiritual mothers posted a quote on Facebook alongside a photograph of bright yellow flowers, much appreciated during a long, frozen February: "I find the great thing in this world is not so much where we stand, as in the direction we are moving: To reach the port of heaven, we must sail sometimes with the wind and sometimes against it—but we must sail, and not drift, nor lie at anchor."[167] We were created to know joy, and even in our fallen state, with effort, we may return to a joyous state of being:

> [J]oy is the final goal, and asceticism is merely the means to achieve it. God likes pleasure; that is why He made it. All the pleasures God made, small and great, are His gifts to us. We don't deserve any of them, and yet God continues daily to pour out His evidently endless cascade of blessing and beauty. And all of it free.[168]

Joy is one emotion, but a life that is becoming prayer endures all things, good and bad, with the act of turning to God. Prayer reflects my relationship with God, and my life becomes a witness of faith. The Saints' prayers help me to learn the way to pray. The words in a prayer book, when I apply them directly to life, are living, and they help me to develop my understanding of God, when I pay attention. As a word-loving convert to the Faith, I initially chose a number of prayers from the prayer book I received when we visited our first Orthodox parish. It was years before I realized that there was a more orthodox rule of prayers for morning, noon, and night. Usually a Christian in the Faith establishes a rule of prayer with the parish priest, and prayer is said to be the first discipline enacted once a person chooses to serve God. The Church provides her people with routine prayer[169] so that, as time allows, one may pray, and prayer can become the center of one's lens on life. Ultimately, so that prayer becomes one's life.

Prayer is a state of mind that includes God—an open mind and heart to Who He is. Importantly, prayer is "not a relaxation exercise but a path to be in communion with [...] God."[170] St. Isaac the Syrian says that one draws near to God by unceasing prayer. Theologians talk about this in-depth, but to me it simply means that God is with me as I go about the day, and I want to see Him in the course of each day.

One morning in late winter, I awoke early, nursed the baby, grabbed my workout

---

167 Oliver Wendell Holmes, Sr.

168 Farley, Fr. Lawrence, "Life is Good," St. Nicholas Orthodox Church, Mentor, OH, parish bulletin, 15 Feb. 2015.

169 *Orthodox Prayer*, http://www.orthodoxprayer.org/index.html, 2015, web, 01 Oct. 2015.

170 Braga, Fr. Roman, "'God is Always With You,' An Interview with Father Roman Braga," http://wonder.oca.org/2012/05/29/god-is-always-with-you-an-interview-with-father-roman-braga/, OCA, 29 May 2012, web, 01 June 2015.

shorts, and headed downstairs. I signed the cross sleepily over the closed doors where the others slept and descended the stairs. Half-way down, I paused in horror. The front door was wide open to the dark morning. I closed and locked the door against a strong breeze and inched about, fearful that someone or something could be in the house. Aware of the possibilities of unwanted intrusion, I began to consider how the Holy Spirit discerns and protects us from unholy spirits, like a strong door against the dark. The Holy Spirit preserves life and enables inner prayer: *Lord Jesus Christ, Son of God, have mercy on me, a sinner.* Life tears at the door of my heart, but in faith, I pray.

Prayer is not a formula; it is a process of wanting to meet with God, personally, deeply. Knowing how to pray is important, but even more crucial is desiring to pray. Wanting to pray sometimes comes of its own accord. In such moments, I have wept, and the prayer has been the closest to Love. When the heart is moved, then God reveals Himself. I think of Abraham, Moses, and the Mother of God who were so close to God. It is beneficial to have role models to inspire us to serve the Lord. The Saints in heaven do more than inspire, they intercede for us, adding their prayers to one's own meager efforts. When a friend is diagnosed with cancer and asks me to pray, I do. The Saints, already where Jesus Christ is, are great helps when it comes to prayer. With the Saints in heaven and others who have faith in God here and now, the cold abandonment of this world is absorbed into the warmth and eternal power of Christ. As St. Seraphim of Sarov says,

> God is a fire that warms and kindles the heart and inward parts. Hence, if we feel in our hearts the cold which comes from the devil - for the devil is cold - let us call on the Lord. He will come to warm our hearts with perfect love, not only for Him but also for our neighbor, and the cold of him who hates the good will flee before the heat of His countenance.[171]

In *The Ladder of Divine Ascent*[172], John Climacus argues that a person who prays must be merciful. He continues, the result of true prayer in one's heart is a flame of love in the soul—realized on earth in some special moments, and in heaven where all moments will be without earthly cares. He says that a person's prayer should be completed for the fullness of spiritual satisfaction, which is of utmost importance because one may not again have the chance to pray for the remission of sins. Climacus warns, "[b]y blurting out one careless word, he who has tasted prayer often defiles his mind, and then when he stands in prayer he no longer attains his desire as before." With an unloving snap to a child, my heart cools, and praying before our meal is perfunctory. When I control my frustration and remain calm, I am able to pray, and to extend a miraculous (if you've dined with small children you understand) peace to those at the table.

---

171 "The Christian Spiritual Life – St. Seraphim," http://www.roca.org/OA/2/2b.htm, Orthodox America, 1980, web, 01 May 2015.
172 Climacus, John, "Prayer is the Mother of Virtues" chapter four in *The Ladder of Divine Ascent,* Paulist Press, 1982.

Changes in me depend on whether I'm feeding my good or bad dog, and they are as twins in me, pawing for "food." A child needs to be taught about these inner dogs. My boys are especially given to video games. My younger son will awake at 6:30, and the next thing I know, he's playing a game. He'll brush his teeth, "After breakfast, Mom!" say a prayer later; make his bed when the covers aren't so impossibly twisted, he promises. The war with him to do what he should, and not what he wants, can begin so early and feel so long in the course of the day. After an especially trying weekend, ending in baby-vomit down my shirt and very little sleep, Monday came as though shot from a canon. My husband took the toddler to a mandatory doctor's appointment to have a medical form signed for her pre-school. My husband and I were both distraught over the intense emotional war parents have to endure when they do not vaccinate their children and well-meaning others do not understand the many reasons why. On this Monday, my worked-up husband came back from the doctor's with our toddler who needed her snack, the first-time ill infant was in my arms as I researched homeopathic cell salts for a fever, the boys were hungry for lunch, and I really just needed to use the restroom. Once I settled the family into lunch, my boys were excited from too much time in the house. They dramatized shooting at each other, and one said, "kill the dead person." I lost it. With the ferociousness of my warring dogs, I tried to explain that we each have twin dogs inside of us. The boys were not allowed to play games where they shot at other people. Period. My son asked if when he turned 18 and moved out of the house he could. I said that I would have no way of controlling that, but for now, they would not. Period.

It is important to teach children that we each have a good and bad dog inside; it is a fight for one, and against another, that creates tension within us. Children may begin to understand the struggle, their own and their parents', and it draws them to perceive the spiritual warfare that we really are engaged in. Each person may become transfigured, transformed into something more beautiful and elevated. Fr. Steven Kostoff writes of Christ's Transfiguration as "A Feast of Divine Beauty."[173] He says, "As human beings created according to the image and likeness of God, we are actually 'images of the Image.' What Christ is, by nature, is what we are meant to be by grace – 'partakers of the divine nature' (1 Peter 1:4)." I pray that I fulfill my responsibility to show my children some degree of self-control that permits them to see my own transfiguration—that is, despite yelling my head off in moments when I lose control. Christ's Transfiguration on Mount Tabor revealed His obedience to God the Father, and the Apostles were able to discern Christ's divine nature, which always was, because of their obedience to God. Obedience is key to effect positive change in my life.

Climacus says that the act of prayer produces different effects in people, but it should always cause change, or the prayer was performed by the body but not the spirit. "If a body is changed in its activity from contact with another body, then how can he remain

---

173 Kostoff, Fr. Steven, "A Feast of Divine Beauty," http://oca.org/reflections/fr.-steven-kostoff/a-feast-of-divine-beauty, OCA, 30 July 2015, web, 01 Aug. 2015.

unchanged who touches the body of God with innocent hands? [...] For prayer is a devout coercion of God." The demons will not waste their time against one who prays continually to God. When a person is obedient and prays, Climacus says that God teaches one how to pray. As is said across the world in an everyday Orthodox Christian prayer: "Pray Lord Thyself in me." When God is present in my life, praying inside of me, than I am naturally transfigured into the image and likeness of Him Who made me. If my life is becoming prayer, I choose to allow this process.

CHAPTER 6
Ancient Christian Prayer, Beyond "Christian Yoga"

Secular spirituality commonly recognizes healing occurs through one's body-mind-spirit.[174] Today, many are spiritual, but asked if they are Christian and spiritual, many wouldn't conclude that they are. To be Christian has come to mean that one knows the Bible and follows Jesus. Of course, this is essential to Christianity, but ancient Christian prayer is highly spiritual and deeply engaging of body-mind-spirit. The head of this life-long endeavor of prayerfulness is God Himself.

I'm exhausted by ten at night, and my evening prayers can lead me into sleep—literally. I aim to pray more in the morning, but Facebook is sometimes a distraction. (It doesn't help that I have placed an app for FB and Scripture side-by-side on my I-phone.) A friend from high school, now a yoga instructor, posts pictures and videos of her amazing body yoga-ing. She includes thoughts and quotes that reflect her sensitive spirit. In a caption to her handstand, body a beautiful arc against morning light through the window of a hotel, she states: Yoga away from home, and I am home.

Home is the experience of realizing who I am created to be and becoming that individual through the grace and love of God. Like my friend, also in her later thirties, I have lived in a number of different places at this point in life: from college days in dorms, apartments, and for a semester abroad in Russia, to living in a small house with Russian in-laws, in a castle on a hill with host-parents, and now a home of our own with four small children. Prayer has always been my "home." I find a quiet place in the pre-dawn morning, usually a vacant bathroom, and I am "home." Through prayer, and all that goes with that quiet, alone time: reflection, planning, (picking-up after boys who ate late after hockey) I am found in meeting with God. Prayer can occur anytime and anywhere, but this special uninterrupted time is a particularly coveted experience of "home" that helps soften my endless earthly cares. When a kid gets up too early, or the husband, I have to really pray for help not to go bananas in my heart for the loss of this essential-to-my-life time.

Prayer to God and meditation are both concerned with deeper, truer understanding of one's self, but the inner content of prayer differs because it is centered on God, and seeking Him helps me understand my own life. Reading scripture and the lives of the Saints points me in the direction of holiness that my own heart cannot get on its own. I desire wellness that is wholeness and holiness, which develops through prayer.

---

174 Cassani, Monica, "The Body/Mind/Soul Can Heal Itself," GreenMedInfo, Blog Entry, http://www.greenmedinfo.com/blog/bodymindsoul-can-heal-itself?page=2, 30 Nov. 2015, web, 30 Nov. 2015.

Christianity differs from meditation in one important way: prayer is communication with God, and meditation is self-focus. Prayer also helps me know myself, but through the lens of Jesus Christ. Meditation may include focus on God, but oftentimes does not. Many today, my friend included, are drawn to Buddhism and Hinduism that use yoga to express the relationship between the body and spirit. Soothing the five senses through stretching, incense, calming music, and comforting words is good. Prayer also effects the body, and the Church appeals to the senses. In a group on Facebook called "The Healing Project", a friend shared an article on the healing properties of frankincense and myrrh. Many in the group, myself included, found this information new. While some had not experienced the aroma of these fine spices, I thought of how the Church has always used them as incense, and how beautifully and perfectly healing Liturgy is. It is said that incense is a strong urging for prayer, and that incense is a holy mystery. My priest said that heaven will be Liturgy. In this life and the next, one has the opportunity to draw unto the merciful Lord as He has always intended, as sung in the Cherubic Hymn: "Let us, who mystically represent the cherubim and sing the thrice-holy hymn to the life-giving Trinity, lay aside all worldly cares, that we may receive the King of all, invisibly escorted by the angelic hosts. Alleluia, alleluia, alleluia."

While there are secular and religious spiritual exercises that help heal the body and spirit, only prayer, as synergy with Christ, is uniquely saving and eternal. Archimandrite Sophrony explains the important difference between true prayer and other meditative endeavors:

It is imperative to draw a very definite line between the Jesus Prayer and every other ascetic theory. He is deluded who endeavors to divest himself mentally of all that is transitory and relative in order to cross some invisible threshold, to realize his eternal origin, his identity with the Source of all that exists; in order to return and merge with Him, the Nameless transpersonal Absolute. Such exercises have enabled many to rise to supra-rational contemplation of being; to experience a certain mystical trepidation; to know the state of silence of the mind, when mind goes beyond the boundaries of time and space. In such-like states, man may feel the peacefulness of being withdrawn from the continually changing phenomena of the visible world; may even have a certain experience of eternity. But the God of Truth, the Living God, is not in all this. It is man's own beauty, created in the image of God, that is contemplated and seen as Divinity, whereas he himself still continues within the confines of his creatureliness.[175]

---

175 Sophrony, Archimandrite, "The Jesus Prayer: Method," http://beforeitsnews.com/christian-news/2013/10/the-jesus-prayer-method-by-archimandrite-sophrony-2484080.html, Before It's News, 08 Oct. 2013, web, Mar., 2015.

Yoga is said to offer a host of benefits. In a recent article[176], the *Natural Society* claims the following benefits: increased strength, agility, and flexibility; improved memory and cognition; weight management; pain reduction; efficient respiratory system; normalized blood pressure; mental health (lessening of anxiety, a sense of well-being and self-actualization, as well as motivation); prevention of degenerative diseases; strengthening of parasympathetic nervous system; and yoga is convenient and can be done anywhere. To be sure, there are many benefits to yoga. This article asserts such bodily benefit that it can seem yoga is a sort of elixir against death. However, unlike prayer that unites one with Christ eternally, yoga is merely a bodily exercise. The meditative state, stretching, and muscle building is good for the body, but against death is helpless. Prayer unites one to the Savior of all.

In Orthodoxy, the body and spirit pray, but the Jesus Prayer is not a Christian yoga. Archimandrite Sophrony discusses how "Lord Jesus Christ, Son of God, have mercy on me a sinner" differs from transcendental meditation. He claims that every culture (not only religious cultures) is concerned with ascetic exercises. Prayer is about freeing one's self "by the power of God from the domination of passions" because Jesus is the only Savior, and His Name evokes actual prayer.

Both yoga and prayer can be spiritual and physical disciplines, but prayer is more than what I can do with my body and in my mind. Prayer centers me in Jesus Christ by the effort I make to say His name, acknowledge His presence, and believe that He is God of my life. This prayerful effort is work, and it changes me from the inside out. My attitude concerning myself, God, and all others changes when I pray. Yoga and other secular meditation practices can strengthen the body, and the mind benefits from self-control and calming of one's thoughts. While such activities are quite helpful for holistic health, a relationship with God distinguishes prayer from other sorts of meditation practices by the essential goal of salvation. Prayer is good for the body and mind, and it profits the soul. By prayer one is saved. St. John of Kronstadt says,

> A man becomes spiritual insofar as he lives a spiritual life. He begins to see God in all things, to see His power and might in every manifestation. Always and everywhere he sees himself abiding in God and dependent on God for all things. But insofar as a man lives a bodily life, and he lives for doing bodily things, he doesn't see God in anything, even in the most wondrous manifestations of His Divine power. In all things, he sees body, material, everywhere and always.[177]

---

176 Sarich, Christina, "Ten Really Amazing Health Benefits of Yoga" http://naturalsociety.com/10-amazing-health-benefits-of-yoga/ Natural Society, 29 Apr. 2015, web, 01 June 2015.

177 Kronstadt, St. John of, *My Life in Christ, or Moments of Spiritual Serenity and Contemplation, or Reverent Feeling, of Earnest Self-Amendment and Peace in God,* Holy Trinity Publications, 2000.

Throughout the ages, prayer has been a physical experience in the Divine Liturgy[178] of the Orthodox Church. This primary prayer service is two-part: the Liturgy of the Word[179], including the reading of Scripture, and the Liturgy of the Eucharist[180], in which the gifts of bread and wine are offered and consecrated to Christ. In this second part of the service, the faithful partake of the bread and wine in a sacramental experience of Holy Communion. Before the Divine Liturgy begins, the priest blesses five loaves of bread in a service called the Prothesis. These loaves of bread symbolize the five loaves in the wilderness from which Christ fed the masses. The priest cuts out a square of bread called the Lamb from the main loaf (prosphora). It is this portion that is consecrated during Liturgy as the Holy Body of Christ. The priest also removes small particles and places them on a plate in commemoration of the Theotokos, various saints, and the living and departed faithful. The leftover bread (antidoron) is blessed and distributed to all people after Liturgy. The priest also blesses the wine and water and pours them into the chalice, to which he will add warm water after the Holy Spirit is called down[181] to "make us and these gifts truly the body and the blood of our Lord and Savior, Jesus Christ."

This is all a holy mystery, but it is effected through the priest's hands and the parishioners' and priest's prayers. I held my infant before the chalice, carefully keeping her reaching arms against her chest with my arm across her. She opened her mouth and the Body and Blood of Jesus Christ was given to the handmaiden of God, "Tatyana." Unexpectedly, my precious, holy daughter spat out Communion. In shock, my free hand caught the fallen Element, as I mumbled to Father, "I got It." I held my baby in my arms, protected her from loss, and helped her accept God. She was not to blame. In our mutual effort together at the chalice of Christ, we were saving our souls: mother holding babe, Father holding the Gifts, the Saints and angels protecting and helping us to hold on to the spiritual reality of the Divine Liturgy. Without all working integrally together, we could not commune. Without the synergistic efforts of our mutual cooperation in Jesus Christ, the experience was a fail. Only in love and togetherness can we be saved.

I gave a bit back to her and licked my finger, feeling confused by the spiritual and physical reality of the Eucharist. It is easy to think only in terms of the physical and to miss the spiritual dimension of life. How hard it can be, even when at the chalice of the Lord, to realize that becoming holy requires faith in the mystery of the Body and Blood of Jesus Christ. I open my mouth, accept the gift, and close my lips to seal the hole from which I can lose my life. This is why we sing, "In faith and love, draw near," because without a ready, willing, and aware countenance, I may expel God from myself.

178 "Divine Liturgy," http://orthodoxwiki.org/Divine_Liturgy, OrthodoxWiki, 12 Jun. 2014, web, 05 Jun. 2015.
179 This part of the service is also called the Liturgy of the Catechumens (for those individuals preparing to enter the Church through chrismation and or baptism).
180 This part of the service is also called the Liturgy of the Faithful; beforehand, the priest and communicants pray that Christ make the bread and wine His body and blood. This is a mystical experience and cannot be explained rationally, i.e., one is not literally eating Christ, but instead benefiting from the ultimate spiritual food of His mystical Body and Blood. Before this portion of the service, catechumens preparing to enter into the Church may leave.
181 This is called the "epiclesis."

The Divine Liturgy is more than a church service that includes soothing music and deep meditative prayer. It is an experience of entering into the Divine, even while here on earth. In the first part of the Liturgy, the priest exclaims: "Blessed is the kingdom of the Father and of the Son and of the Holy Spirit, now and ever and unto ages of ages." After this Rite of Entrance, the Great Litany begins with prayers for the world: peace and salvation, the Church, her bishops, her faithful, captives and their health and salvation, and deliverance from anger and need. It is concluded, as with most litanies, with remembrance of the Theotokos and the Saints. In light of that powerful witness, the faithful are charged to commend their lives to our Lord Jesus Christ. There is a cycle of three prayers and then the "Little Entrance" where we sing: "O Come, let us worship and fall down before Christ. O Son of God... save us who sing to Thee: Alleluia!" At this point, the people have entered the church and gathered around the Word, and common prayers are chanted.

The next portion of the service is understood as rites of proclamation, and Scripture is announced with a psalm and responsive singing. Then, a reader proclaims the epistle or the Acts of the Apostles. The reader's voice is low until the end of the reading when it rises, symbolizing how the early Church rose up from catacombs, the place where the first martyrs were buried. The people sing alleluia and the Gospel is read next. After this, the priest gives a homily, which is a brief reflection on the particular commemorations for the day. Afterwards, there are prayers of supplication and responses of "Lord, have mercy." At the end of this part of the service, the catechumens are prayed for and the people remember the Great Commission to go into the world with the good news of Christ.

The Liturgy of the Faithful opens with the great entrance and the cherubic hymn, or a song of the angels. The priest may then make a procession with the bread and wine, before calling down the Holy Spirit to mystically make it the Body and Blood of Christ. My priest said placing the Elements on the altar reminds him that our lives are laid on the altar as a sacrifice to God. At this point, the Church professes its common faith by reciting the Creed. The liturgical name for this creed is the "Symbol of Faith," indicating its importance to early Christians in determining the orthodoxy of persons claiming to be of the Church. Following the Creed, the priest begins the anaphora, the great Eucharistic prayer over the gifts, so called because of the initial phrase: "Let us lift up our hearts." The people, led by the prayers of the priest, recall the history of the fall and redemption and invoke the Holy Spirit. Having invoked the Holy Spirit and consecrated the gifts, the priest commemorates the Saints, beginning with the Theotokos. At this point, the assembled faithful chant the ancient hymn in honor of the Virgin, "It is truly meet to bless you, O Theotokos, ever-blessed and most pure, and the Mother of our God. More honorable than the cherubim, beyond compare more glorious than the seraphim, without corruption you gave birth to God, the Word. True Theotokos, we magnify you." After consecrating the gifts, commemorating the saints, and praying for the local bishop, the priest lifts up the consecrated gifts, exclaiming, "The holy things are for the holy!" To which the faithful respond, "One is holy, one is Lord, Jesus Christ, to the glory of God the

Father, amen."

The Divine Liturgy is full of body and spirit unity, beginning with the central notion that Christians partake of the Body and Blood of Christ through a mystical reality. The body prays by bowing, censing incense throughout the sanctuary, and revering icons of the Saints. The Saints that have passed on are invisibly and spiritually among those present. Prayer from the mouth is meditation from the heart, without distinction between the body and spirit. As the faithful partake of Holy Communion, people sing the hymn, "O taste and see how good the Lord is." As the Lord is taken into one's own body, this goodness is both physical (we've been fasting and the bread and wine is literally good) and spiritual. I keep the Eucharist in my mouth and stand before the icon of the Theotokos, praying without words, my heart begging for her help. There is a pause before entering back into community when I have "mystically stepped out." Sometimes I feel nothing. Sometimes I feel something. The act is good and helps me believe. Faith, and the prayer that develops with faith, is completely physical, and it is completely spiritual. Prayer merges my life with God's, and all others who also will for Him.

One late afternoon in early spring, I stopped over a friend's home with my daughters. Her young son greeted us incognito, growling like an animal and drawing us into his play. The home was open and incense filled the air. My friend's blue eyes smiled, her feminine laugh drawing us to tea and conversation. We were both new to the neighborhood, drawn to one another by more than a shared interest in wellness of spirit and body. She gently spoke with clarity and confidence. Her humility attracted me. She had suffered a drastic decline in her health that doctors hadn't been able to diagnose. At one point, when she wasn't able to walk up the stairs and mental fog was increasing, when doctors were considering if she had multiple sclerosis, she prayed with her whole heart for God to help her. There seemed nothing to do and no way to understand her suffering, and she gave her life over to God's care. Shortly after, she viewed an advertisement for Celiac's Disease and realized the symptoms described matched some of her's. She changed her diet with an elimination of gluten. Some of her health issues improved.

Faith increased because of her suffering, cry to God, and God's personal response to her. She continued to seek wellness and pray. This was natural to her; she had always been conscious of the spiritual. Even when doctors found a suspicious tumor, with faith and hope, and after her own research, she decided to fight against the odds outside of traditional chemotherapy and radiation. She uses food as medicine and researches natural approaches to wellness, such as essential oils, healing herbs, clean living, and balanced exercise and sleep. She seems well, though she has yet to return to doctors for a diagnosis. My friend's faith in God is central in her life. I am challenged by faith like hers because it isn't called "Orthodox." She wore a cross, and she had Buddhist sayings around her home. She didn't speak of religion, but her love of God was felt. It was felt by a sense of her loving me, loving her son, loving plants and life itself. Love was an energized patience in her. I realized I could not judge her soul, that one could not know another's innermost faith, and the knowledge of this sent chills down my spine.

Life experiences are opportunities where God reveals Himself to individuals. Many times, God's ways are mysterious, and if the heart is open to Truth, He comes with unexpected encounters. There is a sliding glass-door in my kitchen upon which I have suctioned a hanging cross. One morning, I was opening the drapes and thought that I smelled church. I leaned closer to the curtains before the cross, and there was a slight fragrance. God's revelations are unexpected and come by faith. Faith is in the heart, and it may sound silly to put words to experiences that develop one's personal faith. The sky is more majestic than the fragrance on my drapes, and yet how unnoticed it sometimes goes.

Experiences in life reveal God to each of us, if we are open to knowing Him as He really is. When my priest said that heaven will be Liturgy, I asked about those for whom Liturgy is not their church experience. In humility, my priest simply said that we cannot try to understand God's mercy on this side of the Kingdom of Heaven, but God said that when two or more are gathered He is present. This "gathering" wasn't ever intended to be at a coffee shop with each one's own interpretation of the Bible. There was always a liturgical structure to worship, a Holy Tradition, which keeps order and prevents chaos, schism, and error. Worship of God is not something one makes up but something one learns, passes down through the generations, and by which one is saved.

Baptism is a family's choice to set an infant's life along a path, in the Church, so that that child will have regular opportunities to encounter God through the life of the Church. Growing up Protestant, I hadn't understood the tradition of baptizing infants. At this earlier time in my life, I had thought baptism was a symbol of a person's faith, and a baby couldn't yet decide what it believed. Now, I see baptism as the promise it is to raise an infant in the Holy Tradition of Christ's Church so that when the child is older, he or she will not depart from it. The Church welcomes all who come with the hope that each will choose to follow Christ by repentance and the Holy Sacraments.

The Body of Christ, the Church, is more than a place with walls and carpet. It is the living, loving members of Jesus Christ, who are meant to share the truth and power of God by our very lives. Baptism is entrance into relationship with all others also living in Christ. When our fourth child was baptized and the priest cut her hair, my grandmother asked what he was doing. The priest tonsures a newly baptized person as one's very first sacrifice to God. From what one has been given, one gives, beginning with the body and extending to all gifts in this life. The hair is an important symbol as a part of the body itself that is given to God when a babe is 40 days old. A family together recognizes the spiritual reality when it vows to raise a child in Christ. Though a child does not understand it, she experiences the Eucharist, the anointing of healing oils, and the prayers against Satan and his minions. As a person grows and continues experiencing the Faith: services of the church, community with other believers and shared life-events, and personal prayers throughout the day within a cycle of feasts and fasts and commemoration of the Saints, understanding increases for life in Christ. It is a wonder that some parents today give so many lesser experiences to their children and haven't the time for the most important gift of the Faith. Regular Holy Communion builds our bodies and feeds our souls in mysterious and practical ways.

The Church rejoices with each baptism because "As many as have been baptized into Christ, have put on Christ. Alleluia."[182] At Orthodox Christian baptisms, we hymn that the baptized "put on Christ." Fr. Morelli explains that putting on Christ in the modern world is to continue the ascetic practices of our Spiritual Fathers[183]:

> If we put on Christ at baptism and continue to wash ourselves through repentance, then we are able to reflect the light of Christ. Our constant prayer is, 'Lord Jesus Christ, Son of God, have mercy on me a sinner.' We are creatures. We have no independent existence. We depend on God for all and by his mercy, we can have the light of Christ indwell in us. This is a spiritual reality revealed by Our Lord Jesus Christ Himself. The value of this is unfathomable.[184]

Protestant Christians say that they are "born again," and for the Orthodox, through the sacrament of baptism, the old person dies in the font and rises again in new life. Baptism into Christ initiates a life-long process of developing one's life as a prayer through a personal relationship with Christ. Baptismal prayers funnel life into a Christian matrix that is preserved and protected from heresy by the teachings of the Holy Catholic and Apostolic Church. Through the sacrament, one is covered with prayers against the evil one and his unholy spirits that make their "lair in the heart." Father says, "Depart from this newly enlisted warrior of Christ," because one who is baptized in Jesus Christ is protected from the unseen principalities who aim to draw each one to the dark side, against God. Protected, yes, but called to become a "warrior of Christ," which indicates that each person who chooses God has to exert effort and carry his unique cross in this life. In this way, a person accepts salvation that the Lord died to grant each of us.

A friend and I enjoyed an afternoon of watermelon and corn-on-the-cob as the seven children between us played and bounced with energy. As I was loading up the minivan and leaving, she leaned in to me and lamented that her newborn would have to suffer life in our fallen, troubled world. "My friend," I thought so naturally, on this good day, "this world is God's creation. When He returns, all that is imperfect will be made right." It was easy to sense the good in the world as I looked up at the summer sky, her wide green lawn and the huge trees about us like promises of strength and eternity. Her sentiment came from thoughts of others who were not free and safe. She asked if I'd heard of the recent slaughter of Christians in Africa. Some didn't see trees or feel summer. This world's suffering was real.

182 Hymned at each Holy Baptism.
183 Morelli, George, *Healing – Volume 1: Orthodox Christianity and Scientific Psychology*, Eastern Christian Publications, 2006, p. 22.
184 Morelli, George, *Healing – Volume 1: Orthodox Christianity and Scientific Psychology*, Eastern Christian Publications, 2006, p. 27.

I thought about my friend's feelings as I drove home. Life could seem bad when hells of this world cornered one. A Christian cleaved to the strength of the Lord, in the good, and in the bad, believing that no matter what, God was loving, real, and would save us in the end. That was amazing and comforted me, but I wasn't in Africa. There is always evil, always sin, and it isn't long before the summer sky gives way to a clap of thunder.

God is in all seasons of life. In the After-feast of Transfiguration, we sing: "The voice of Your thunder was in the whirlwind; Your lightning lighted up the world; the earth trembled and shook. You are clothed with honor and majesty, Who cover Yourself with light as with a garment." God is beyond the light, the air, and the trees. God is more than all of the world and every living thing, and there is no way to meditate my way to Him. By grace, I know God and am known by Him. The living grace of God feeds us. We feed each other with faith in God that helps us see the bigger picture in a moment. There will always be hope, no matter what hells come. In the end, the soft light of summer will reign down upon God's creation.

God is the deepest well of power, love and goodness. Ironically, secular meditations that draw me into myself cannot save me. A self-satisfied attitude won't lead me closer to Truth because I am happy enough staying where I am. When I seek God, I am challenged by His call to love others and be like Him. The Holy Spirit convicts me of my own sins, and if I choose God, then repentance of sins that separate me from Him feels necessary because I long to be in communion with God.

Sometimes, it seems that I would be happier to do what I want, rather than submit to God. Then, I assume a self-justified attitude and prayer. *Lord Jesus Christ, Son of God, have mercy on me a sinner*, begins to seem obsolete. My prayer becomes a sort of meditation on my own needs, thoughts, and words. The difference between self-serving meditation and genuine prayer is Jesus Christ in my mind and heart. Monk Seraphim says, "Don't criticize or judge other people—regard everyone else as an angel, justify their mistakes and weaknesses, and condemn only yourself as the worst sinner. This is step one in any kind of spiritual life." Archimandrite Sophrony claims:

> In the atmosphere of the world today, prayer requires super human courage. The whole ensemble of natural energies is in opposition. To hold on to prayer without distraction signals victory on every level of existence. The way is long and thorny but there comes a moment when a heavenly ray pierces the dark obscurity to make an opening through which can be glimpsed the source of the eternal Divine Light.

Christ frees one who chooses to obey Him from enslavement of the passions. Temptations are said to remain until one's last breath, but a Christian serves Christ rather than sin. Even though there are no perfect roads and we all sin, turning away from sin once again and towards Christ liberates mankind. Many youth today are frustrated and faithless. More than half of parents (who marry) divorce, and current family life is often very stressful. Outside of the Church, young people have little encouragement to seek faith in the Father, Son, and Holy Spirit. For the most part, cultural role models do not demonstrate obedience to God and love towards others. Instead, with an attitude of self-love, self-worship, and self-as-God, popular figures express bizarre notions of self-worship. Young people today do not often seem drawn to their parents' versions of Christianity, as many of their parents have turned away from faith that hasn't formed roots beyond denominations divided from other denominations. As a result of wanting goodness, even God, but not seeing examples of faith that draw them, young people decide to go their own ways. Many people today make up their own faith systems. They may meditate on their own inner beings and experience illusions of illumination and peace.

A student of mine was very angry as we discussed his essay on fate. The red crawled up his neck, and I was silenced by the struggle I felt in him. He argued that people with faith worry about everything and don't recognize that fate will determine what will be. He didn't like discussing his ideas that hadn't reached conclusions. He thought that those with faith were confident and certain. I later thought of this student's observations of anxiety and pride in those who profess faith in God, and it reminded me that this is not the way to attract people. Certainly, a spirit of peace and humility had drawn me into Orthodoxy.

Faith and faithlessness is a choice, in process throughout one's lifetime. Faith is fluid and salvation, faith, and prayer grow in the heart over the course of one's lifetime. By God's presence in our lives, a person's life is becoming prayer. Archimandrite Sophrony says, "To acquire prayer is to acquire eternity. When the body lies dying, the cry 'Jesus Christ' becomes the garment of the soul; when the brain no longer functions and other prayers are difficult to remember, in the light of the divine knowledge that proceeds from the Name our spirit will rise into life incorruptible."

Many around me talk about centering, meditating, and nurturing spiritual balance in their lives. Some people believe to be a good person and seek self-control via meditation is enough and even better than reliance on the supernatural. The Humanist Community Project claims that "secular meditation"[185] is a response to the stress of life that includes techniques to manage stress, which are free of religion and proselytizing. Through meditation, individuals foster compassion for self and others by clearing the mind and calming emotions. Such meditation is supported by science, the site argues, and has "nothing to do with supernaturalism." Rather, it is a place where "great" supportive people meet together to stretch, breathe, and share personal joys and concerns. "This is the emotional and visceral side of Humanism."

---

185 The Humanist Hub, http://harvardhumanist.org/harvard/humanist-mindfulness-group-mor/, Harvard University, 2015, web, 01 June 2015.

Testimonials posted focus on one's self, disconnected from others, though comments affirm that meditation connects them to others:

> I started reading about Buddhism over the past couple of years, and started my own informal practice, but I couldn't really talk to people at work about it. Then I tried a bunch of Buddhist groups but they often involved altars, or things that felt like praying, or gods, or magical powers...I really like that the Humanist Mindfulness Group is more science-based. I'm not even sure if I'm a Humanist. I know I don't believe in the supernatural, but I'm open to experience different things...still, I figure if I'm going too far towards either rationality or supernaturalism, I'll go with rationality, and this group gives me the opportunity to do that and still meditate with others.

> Meditation opens up new experiences for me; it helps me feel more calm, more aware. I'm an atheist who appreciates that there is a lot of wisdom in the non-Karma, non-reincarnation aspects of Buddhism.

> Meditation helps me be a better teacher, a better family member, a better member of the community.

> Meditation makes me more compassionate, and I think that's what we all need in the 21st century, more compassion.

> I like myself better when I meditate, I have greater empathy. It really makes it easier to understand other people and what they're feeling.

Science and faith are not mutually exclusive. No matter how much one knows, there is always the choice to believe in a particular theory based on evidence interpreted by subjects with ideologies and experiences. It seems to me that our bodies and minds are in a constant circular motion as we meet out our arguments. The mind and body cannot be divided. I understand experiences based on my knowledge frames, and I change my mind when lived experiences show me otherwise. People must open their minds and consider that which challenges assumptions and norms that do not make sense against life experiences. When I have changed, and when I have seen others change, it has been with humility that searches the truth of a situation through prayer that is with reason but beyond it.

Meditation does not rely on communication with God, prayer is only concerned with that—all the rest of my body-spirit discipline is to quiet myself and invite the Holy Spirit into my own. According to Fr. George Morelli, current behavioral research uses the Buddhist philosophy of mindfulness as a clinical tool to break bad habits and troubling emotions. The psychologist Kabat-Zinn[186] explains mindfulness as "awareness that emerges through paying attention on purpose, in the present moment, and non-judgmentally to the unfolding of experience moment by moment." The focus in Buddhism is to attend to the sensory and physical aspects of a moment and to recognize thought patterns, feelings, and physical sensations that occur. When one does, one may learn to tell the difference between thought, emotion, and physical sensations. Then, one may make choices based on what one really wants. Mindfulness can occur in meditative and non-meditative states.

Morelli explains that the early Church Fathers spoke of "nepsis," or vigilance of the mind and heart. This notion is similar to mindfulness and metacognition, or thinking about one's thinking. It is a practice that leads to wellness by reconciling the body and spirit as one, as personhood. To be wakeful and attentive is necessary for prayer, and it is likened to the manner in which a mother pays attention to an infant, or a soldier to others in battle.

Vigilance of my mind takes effort. I often have to re-read a simple prayer so that the words sink into my distracted mind. I have heard it is better to focus and say one prayer, than to read an entire canon in a distracted manner. I have taken this to heart, even on occasions before Liturgy when I haven't found the time to read my full rule, I try to find a quiet corner to say one meaningful prayer, to silence the earthly cares and open to God. There are times when all I offer is a gut-wrenching sigh before entering the doors to the church. I try to then close my eyes, and even this seems a prayer because I am mindful of Jesus Christ. Christians utilize nepsis in prayer to detect harmful habits, to realize emotional reactions that are damaging to one's self and/or others, to choose to be vigilant in mind and body, and to counteract negative responses with prayers that re-route one's heart and mind to goodness.

Morelli says there is an "anthropological and theological chasm" between the ethos of Buddhists' mindfulness and Christians' nepsis because the traditional understanding of mindfulness omits God. The experience of noetic knowledge is beyond one's own mind; it is an encounter with God and the experience of grace poured into the heart. For the Church Fathers, the mind is the "nous" and is located deep in the heart. Morelli writes:

> Thus, mindfulness that is separated from God is never a true Christian mindfulness. The mindful, noetic, mind of a person is enlightened by an illumination from God, through the Holy Spirit, in the depth of the heart and mind, which allows perception of spiritual experience. True and purified reason

---

186 Kabat-Zinn, Jon, "Mindfulness-Based Interventions in Context: Past, Present, and Future," http://www-psych.stanford.edu/~pgoldin/Buddhism/MBSR2003_Kabat-Zinn.pdf, American Psychological Association, 2003, web, 01 Oct. 2015.

will burn more brightly, like a light.[187]

We are on a journey through life, and its end is God—whether we want Him or not. Through prayer, we choose to have a relationship with the Lord throughout our lives. We desire God more, more as our hearts soften to the Creator of all, and prayer becomes our way of life. Secular meditation, so popular today, cannot provide the depth of lasting goodness that I seek. Meditation is good, but the depth of myself is revealed more completely through prayer to God. In a personal relationship with Him, I experience Love: hope, inspiration, and healing.

Christianity is about effort and work, but it all adds up to the greatest joy. A friend posted a video of an Orthodox priest blessing people with water on Pascha. He was showering the place with drenched palms in an energized joy that created sober and glorious laughter among the people. "This Is Orthodoxy." I couldn't agree more.

---

187 Morelli, George, "Mindfulness as Known by the Church Fathers," http://www.antiochian.org/mindfulness-known-church-fathers, Antiochian Orthodox Christian Archdiocese, web, 01 Apr. 2015.

CHAPTER 7
Unavoidable Illness and Death, Our Saving Road

"O Lord, save Your people and bless Your inheritance."[188]

My three year old was impressed with the paradox that God died. We attended Liturgy for the Exaltation of the Precious and Life-giving Cross, and afterwards she continued to ask: "God died?" I would begin a too-theological response, to which she straightforwardly commented, "He loves us so much. He's here with us. He saves me." In his homily during the service, our priest mentioned that there are two colors for priests' vestments in Divine Liturgy for the feast of the Life-giving Cross: red and green. On the one hand, the cross marks death, and blood is appropriate. On the other hand, the cross is a symbol of new life. Christ tramples death by death, and upon those in the tomb, He bestows life. There is no greater mystery than our salvation. Fr. Steven Kostoff[189] writes: "How can suffering and death be the path to glorification and life with God?" He answers this question with the fact that the cross is always linked to the Resurrection of Christ, and so it is both an instrument of suffering and death and a symbol of our glory in Christ's holy resurrection. Fr. Kostoff borrows St. Paul's response: "'For the word of the cross is folly to those who are perishing, but to us who are being saved it is the power of God.'"[190]

The cross was not merely a political symbol, as it stood for life and triumph of the Giver of Life, the Lord, in the fourth century. The cross had been in the dark, literally, awaiting Emperor Constantine. When he brought the Cross to light, he allowed honor and witness of the Christians who had been persecuted beforehand. The Christian people sang: "O Lord, save Thy people and bless Thine inheritance. Grant victory to the Orthodox kings over the barbarians!" This, at the time, Byzantine "national anthem" rightfully attributed to the Cross the spiritual and physical protection of those willing to have faith in God. Fr. Lawrence Farley[191] tells of the history of Christ's cross, how it was buried during the persecution of Christians, unearthed by Constantine, and how it has been again "forced into the cultural catacombs." Nonetheless, the power of the Cross comes from the Holy Spirit, Farley reminds us, and is upon those who suffer for their Master. The Cross is not simply a wooden relic, which can be lost to history. It is disciple's determination to serve the Lord even at the cost of suffering, blood, and death. When reproached for bearing the name 'Christian,' Christ's disciples rejoice and count

188 Psalm 28:9
189 Kostoff, Fr. Steven, "Before Your Cross We Bow Down in Worship," St. Nicholas Church, Mentor, OH, parish bulletin, 13 Sept. 2015.
190 1 Corinthians 1:18
191 Farley, Fr. Lawrence, "Byzantium and the Glory of the Cross," St. Nicholas Church, Mentor, OH, parish bulletin, 20 Sept. 2015.

themselves blessed, for the Spirit of glory and of God rests upon them.[192]

In a correspondence with my spiritual father, he said that Orthodoxy teaches that in this world we will suffer. In our consumeristic culture, many latch onto pharmaceutical promises that we can evade pain and suffering. Taking medication to alleviate pain and suffering is not a sin, and in many cases modern medicine is a blessing to be sure. The deep-seated, tangled-up problem is that pharmaceuticals have side effects that cause suffering, and in the greed for money, lives are being destroyed from within the body. We feel badly, and cleave to our health care, but sometimes it is our very health care that leads us to feel badly in the first place.

While suffering is a given, God does not will for babies to be injected with harmful substances. It seems to me that we are engaged in spiritual warfare that is centered within our very bodies. The evil one actively aims to desecrate the sanctity of life, and he is doing so through pharmaceutical companies, primarily through their campaign to vaccinate everyone, everywhere from the moment they are born until death. In today's western culture, discernment is needed to choose what will actually build the body and feed the spirit. America today is bombarded with advertisements for pharmaceutical promises to feel well; these are often optical illusions when we are not more well in taking the drugs into our bodies. In today's culture, it is difficult to unbraid the ills that harm wholeness and holiness in our lives, but if we do not try, then we will continue to be harmed. It is better to realize the truth of our bodies and spirits and what helps us to be well. Yes, we will suffer and die, and a Christian bears the cross, but life is a gift that we fight to preserve, nurturing wellness of the body and spirit as we are able, and as we are called by God to do.

Concerning spiritual health, Isaac the Syrian says, "The sick one who is acquainted with his sickness is easily to be cured; and he who confesses his pain is near to health. Many are the pains of the hard heart; and when the sick one resists the physician, his torments will be augmented."[193] According to Matt. 12:31, blasphemy of the Holy Spirit is the only unpardonable sin. In the Orthodox Christian Symbol of Faith (creed), we state, "I believe in the Holy Spirit, the Lord, and Giver of Life, Who proceeds from the Father, Who with the Father and the Son together is worshipped and glorified, Who spoke by the Prophets." The Holy Spirit is the Lord Who gives life. It is unpardonable when we "blaspheme," which is to speak evil of God. When we intentionally harm our bodies or others', we blaspheme the Giver of Life. I believe many of our sins in the "collective" body of our nation follow from ignorance, but it is time to become aware of life and death, preserving that which gives life and turning from that which does not. Life and death is for God to give, according to His will.

---

192 1 Peter 4: 14
193 "From Homily Two," *Saint Isaac the Syrian, Quotes from Homilies,*
http://andreaskoutsoudis3.com/orthodox-christian-quotes/saint-isaac-the-syrian-quotes-from-homilies/,
Wordpress blog, 2015, web, 17 Oct. 2015.

Each one is ill and in need of the Physician of Souls. To be made well, a person has to feel the pains of a broken life—to acknowledge the disappointments, hurts, and wrongs that haven't been made right, whether because of one's own actions or the actions of others, and forgive one's self and all others. Healing is a process through repentance and confession, and God's forgiveness of sins saves our souls. The words of the priest's prayer before confession tenderize my broken heart:

> O God our Savior who granted David the King pardon of his sin when he repented before the prophet Nathan; in your overwhelming love for all humans, accept the repentance of these your servants who seek forgiveness for the sins they have committed. Overlook all they have done wrong pardoning their offenses and absolving their iniquities, since you once said Lord: 'I do not want a sinner to die, but rather that he turn from his sin and live:' and 'even to seventy times seven sins should be forgiven!' For your majesty is beyond compare and your mercy is without limit and if you held our sins against us who would stand? But you are the God of those who repent and to you we ascribe glory, to the Father, and to the Son, and to the Holy Spirit now and ever and unto ages of ages. Amen.

Becoming whole and Building Natural Immunity in the Body and Soul is anchored in honoring the sanctity of life. When our lives are becoming prayer, even illness and death are opportunities to express the Holy Spirit and Giver of Life. St. Ignaty Brianchaninov[194] says that the mind of mankind has been so darkened by the fall that we forget death. He says that the Jesus Prayer and remembrance of death merge as one activity, "From the prayer comes vivid remembrance of death, as if it were a foretaste of it: and from this foretaste of death, the prayer itself flares up more vigorously." No matter how many organic apples I eat, or how many afternoon jumping jacks I do, suffering in this world is promised, and mortality is assured.

Just as the cross is an instrument of death and suffering as well as a symbol of resurrection and new life, each of our lives is as a saving road to salvation. The sanctity of life is felt on quiet walks to the lake, prayerful drives to work, and heart-giving prayers in the night. When the new day dawns, Truth rises like the sun in the east and spreads its glorious light. God, the Giver of Life, is everywhere and fills all things. No matter what illness and suffering might accompany the day at hand.

When a person prays throughout life and seeks meaning and purpose in God's plan for her days, perhaps death becomes a fierce prayer of sorts, asking God for mercy and forgiveness and loving Him and all others with each breath. My spiritual Father told a story of an elderly priest who was widowed and lived in a small apartment. They met and shared coffee and cake after Liturgy, and when the elderly man was asked if he was

---

194 Brianchaninov, St. Ignaty, "On the Remembrance of Death," www.orthodoxinfo.com/death/stignaty-death.aspx, Orthodox Christian Information Center, 2015, web, 01 Oct. 2015.

lonely living alone, he simply said that he was not living alone at all. With him always was the Father, Son, and Holy Spirit.

The body may or may not be healed, but even in dying the soul can become more well. We pray each Liturgy for a peaceful death and a good defense before the dread judgement seat of Christ. Stanley Harakas says "eu-thanasia" in Greek means a good death where one's moral and spiritual purity provides a sense of hope and trust in God. In this way, "True humanity may be achieved even on a deathbed." A friend was diagnosed with stomach cancer years ago, and her tiny body withered to less than seventy pounds. She couldn't ingest more than a small pea at a time. Once, I brought her some blessed bread and sat at the edge of her bed. The whites of her eyes were yellow and her teeth appeared so vibrant and white. She sipped water and spoke softly. In her feeble beauty, she recounted that she didn't need to eat, she only wanted to live. She had dreamed that if she continued collecting coins, she could remain alive. She stared into my eyes without flinching, and I couldn't look away. She said that she wanted to plant flowers in the spring. With waning energy, she gathered some clothes for me to take, both of us knowing that there wouldn't be another spring for my friend. I held her hands and we wept to the Mother of God. *Please help my friend let go,* I prayed. "Look with loving-kindness, O all hymned Theotokos, upon my cruel bodily suffering, and heal the sickness of my soul."[195]

Those who perceive the Body of Christ are great encouragements to humanity, in life and in death. In the General Moleben we hymn: "Precious in the sight of the Lord is the death of His saints." In March 2015, 37 year-old Fr. Matthew Baker of CT was killed in an auto accident while driving home from vespers. His five small children, who were also in the car, were unharmed. His wife had been at home recovering from having recently delivered their stillborn child. In the midst of death, this family encouraged the world to have faith in God.

In his lifetime, Fr. Baker had been compared to Georges Florovsky, a 20th century Russian Orthodox priest, theologian, and ecumenist, which is one who aims to unite the Church throughout the world. Florovsky said there are two aspects of religious knowledge: revelation and experience. Philip Dorroll[196] explains, "Religious truth is discursively expressed it terms of human doctrines and the concepts that structure them, but insofar as religious truth refers to the ineffable it cannot be confined by human mental formulations and is experienced through the grace of the divine itself." Florovsky and Baker were concerned with inspiring Christians through lively intellectual debates on the early Church Fathers' teachings rather than intellectual debates on

---

195 From the General Moleben, a service of intercession or supplication.
196 Dorroll, Philip, "Scripture and Dissent: Engaging with Neo-Patristic Paradigm of Modern Orthodox Theology," http://orthodox-theology.com/media/PDF/IJOT2.2013/Dorroll-Scripture-and-Dissent.pdf, *International Journal of Orthodox Theology*, 4:2, 2013, pg. 137.

Scholasticism or Reformation. Florovsky uses the term "Neo-Patristic Synthesis" to mean application of the teachings of the Church in current times with life experiences. Fr. Baker argued that most of the seminal works of Orthodox dogma and theology throughout the centuries had actually not been ruminations on established texts and practices but theological and philosophical challenges offered by the non-Orthodox.

It is important to know others, to listen to what they think and feel and why, and care deeply for the world. This doesn't necessarily mean that I must agree with others, but I understand myself in relationship with other people. For example, the more I reflect on the world's many ways of spiritualizing the body's emotional and physical needs through yoga, secular meditation, and Prozac, the more I realize the central place of prayer. Life in Christ is the fulfillment of an in-born need and life-long desire for cosmic order, goodness, and beauty. When life is becoming prayer, purple flowers are not just beautiful, they are also meaningful and purposeful—beyond their place in an ecosystem, as also an expression of life and truth given to us by our Creator.

My eight-year-old son and his friend debated whether God chooses "us" or we choose Him. My son was adamant with a simple yet meaningful point: *God wouldn't just kick us down*, he continued to say to his friend, drawing me in with, *right, mom?* I left the dishes in the sink and joined their conversation, which had paused their Mine-craft video game. *You are both right*, I began, explaining that God chooses each of His creations when He allows life. It is each one's choice to accept God or to reject Him. Acceptance of God relates one's entire life to God, and in the course of a lifetime, all things are understood as being in relationship to God. If a person does not wish to see his life in relationship to God, God allows for that. In such cases, when faced with God, one would not desire His love, the experience would burn, as though searing into a heart not on fire for the Lord of all. The Orthodox Church teaches that each one's reception of God is what Scripture means by the Kingdom of Heaven is within you. We choose to grow in a personal relationship with God, or we choose not to. Depending on a relationship we've developed with God through prayer and good works, upon death, we uniquely experience "heaven" or "hell."

The Church is alive through the very particular life experiences of everyday people who will for God and have accepted the unbroken ancient line of Orthodox Christianity. Each one's life is meant to tell a rich anecdote in the global tale of Love spanning across time. St. Nicholas of Serbia says, "Truth is not a thought, not a word, not a relationship between things, not a law. Truth is a Person. It is a Being, which exceeds all beings and gives life to all. If you seek truth with love and for the sake of love, she will reveal the light of His face to you inasmuch as you are able to bear it without being burned."[197]

---

197 "Thoughts on Good and Evil," http://orthodox.cn/patristics/300sayings_en.htm, *Three-hundred Sayings of the Ascetics of the Orthodox Church*, Ven. Serapion Kozheozersky, ed., Moscow, Orthodox Missionary Society, 2011, web, 01 June 2015.

My aunt was passing away with breast cancer when I was full-blown pregnant with our second daughter. I visited her in the hospital and read her a prayer for the dying. She asked me to repeat it to her, "It gives me comfort," she whispered. I nestled close to her shallow breath and spoke softly. I felt her warm hand as the sound of life rose and fell between us. There was so much life between us. I didn't know what kind of young mother she had been or what her youth had been like. I knew that she had taken me to the library and to second-hand stores for shopping when I was just out of college. I loved her, and felt close to her. Death itself is a prayer, perhaps a final prayer, as we fall asleep in the Lord.

It's worth wondering what sort of witness my life is to those around me. Protopresbyter Thomas Hopko[198] recently died. Just before Pascha, three nuns from a neighboring monastery visited him. They were welcomed warmly by Fr. Hopko's wife, and they took the decorated Cross from the monastery chapel and sang hymns and prayed with the family. They sang hymns of Holy Week, and one of the Mothers read the 17th chapter of St. John's Gospel near his ear. "Father, breathing calmly and quietly, eyes always closed, seemed to react to all this in the very slightest but clear ways: raising his eyebrows with slight mouth movements during the singing." They asked that the Lord shine His face upon Fr. Hopko.

In his writing on death[199], Fr. Hopko claims that mankind is created for life, and that it is not God's will that we die. Death is the enemy, as the Apostle Paul calls death the "last enemy." Fr. Hopko says, "Death is not natural [...] and not willed by God. [...] Death comes into the world as a rebellion against God. Death comes into the world because people do not choose life, but choose death, darkness, and themselves over God." He explains that the demons, as lovers of death, darkness, and evil, draw us to death. One counters this draw to death by obedience to God. We each die, but Fr. Hopko argues we would not if we always listened and obeyed God, impossible in this fallen world.

Fr. Hopko explains that God didn't kill Adam and Eve for eating fruit. Rather, by their personal choice to defy God and disobey, they "committed suicide." Further, we have passed along this "ancestral sin" to our children through the ages—it is a self-will to do what is outside of God's will.

[T]he human task is to overcome and destroy death, and to make death to die so that life can then live. The problem, however, is that in our time death has been so naturalized nobody will even think of it as an enemy. In much literature, it is considered the last stage of life, normal, or you go into some sort of light somewhere, and if you are tired of this life or this world, you call some doctor to end your life. However, for Biblical Christians, that is absolutely not

---

198 Dean Emeritus of Saint Vladimir's Orthodox Theological Seminary, Crestwood, NY, and noted Orthodox Christian priest, theologian, and speaker.
199 Hopko, Fr. Thomas, "Life after death... Mysteries beyond the grave," http:www.orthodoxchristian.info/pages/afterdeath.htm, Oct. 1999, Brisbane, Australia, web, 01 Oct. 2015.

the teaching.

He compares the deaths of Socrates and Jesus. Socrates corrupted the youth of Athens arguing that one who could face death was a true philosopher. He was put to death with hemlock and drinks it willfully. On the other hand, Jesus sweats blood and prays to His Father for the cup to be taken from Him, though He accepts His Father's will. To die is an outrage; "it is the total victory of the devil. We were created to sing hallelujah to God, not to be corrupted and rot in the tomb." But Jesus accepts His Father's will in perfect harmony as God.

Jesus's friend Lazarus dies to show the truth of God's love that conquers even death. John 11:3-4 states, "Therefore the sisters sent to Him, saying, 'Lord, behold, he whom You love is sick.' When Jesus heard that, He said, 'This sickness is not unto death, but for the glory of God, that the Son of God may be glorified through it.' Jesus weeps at the death of his friend, He groans in his spirit for the sorrow of loss, shared with Lazarus' sisters. Mary says that she knows whatever Christ asks the Father will be granted, and by her faith Lazarus awakens and rises. It was God's will to show that death is conquered by faith and love through Jesus Christ. This event prefigures the Passion of Christ, and Christians celebrate this historical event two weeks before Pascha. Christ responds to death with fear and sadness and with acceptance and faith in the plan of salvation, that conquers even death. When Lazarus dies, Christ weeps. There is genuine mourning and a process of grief before Lazarus is risen. This is the way for us, as well. Celebrations of life come at the resurrection, not in restaurants here on earth shortly after one's passing. In a grave sense, denying death removes the deeper meaning of life.

When we fail to realize death, we cannot understand the meaning of life as the antithesis of death. People have always misunderstood death. In the Old Testament, the Sadducees believed that death was natural and one went to be with loved ones. To the Sadducees, God lived on in the people of Israel. They did not believe that one had a spirit, and they did not believe that those who died would be resurrected from the dead. The Pharisees understood the Scriptures and believed in the soul, the resurrection, and the Messianic age. The Pharisees believed that with the resurrection, God's glory would fill creation and His kingdom would be established on earth: graves would open, the dead would rise, and all who have ever lived would be judged.

So the Light of Israel will be for a fire, and his Holy One for a flame; it will burn and devour His thorns and his briers in one day. And it will consume the glory of his forest and of his fruitful field, both soul and body; and they will be as when a sick man wastes away. Then the rest of the trees of his forest will be so few in number that a child may write them. And it shall come to pass in that day that the remnant of Israel, and such as have escaped of the house of Jacob, will never again depend on him who defeated them, but will depend on the Lord, the Holy One of Israel, in truth.[200]

Fr. Hopko explains that there is no hell until the end of time. Those who fall asleep in the Lord, pass into the hands of God and He cares for them. This "blissful state of death" is called the bosom of Abraham:

If you have even been to an Orthodox funeral, you hear the fifth chapter of St. John's gospel. It says, '... the hour is coming in which all who are in the grave will hear His voice and come forth - those who have done good, to the resurrection of life, and those who have done evil, to the resurrection of condemnation. I can of Myself do nothing. As I hear, I judge; and My judgement is righteous, because I do not seek My own will but the will of the Father who sent Me.' This part of the gospel is extremely important, which says all and everyone will be raised. Not just the good people, but everyone. This Universal Resurrection is our teaching, because death is destroyed.

Fr. Thomas Hopko fell asleep in the Lord on March 18, 2015 at three in the afternoon. His memory is alive in my heart, may it be eternally in our Lord's. I think of his life and realize that prayer is more than words in the morning or before bed. His life showed his family and many others the Faith. Prayer is one's entire life. Each has different talents, but God has intentionally created each one with attributes that would increase good in the world.

In Pascha, we hymn, "Your resurrection, O Christ our God, the angels in heaven sing, enable us on earth, to worship you in purity of heart." The Church, created from the beginning of time and established with Christ, continues as a gift of grace that the Holy Spirit reveals to us in our very lives. Presvytera Vassi Haros states, "The Church, under the protection and guidance of Orthodoxy, is tangible and spiritual. The body and soul realize each other in the sacraments, prayer, charity, etc. and this should be happening all the time." The Church is from God, and it is the Body of Christ. "When You, O Lord, were baptized in the Jordan, the Trinity was made manifest. And the Spirit, in the form of a Dove, confirmed the truthfulness of Your Word." Each one baptized into Christ is called to live out faith. This lived faith is prayer.

On Good Friday, my daughter called from her highchair. "I come church!" I hadn't planned on taking the smallest ones, but the joy in her request confirmed she'd come, too. The sanctuary was somber but bone-chillingly beautiful: thick incense dark and crimson, Christ in the tomb—symbolically represented under a sheet of glass where a knit icon depicting his body was kissed: His shoulders, the Word—placed atop the center of the glass, His feet. So cold against my lips. Eyes closed to my children, to the parishioners, the world shutout for shaky moments with a literal feeling of being sucked into another realm. *Ideas are in the way of the experience of Love.* Out, again. My son asked, how much longer is service? I held the baby against me and breathed deeply, taking in the spiritual reality that alone would fuel the spirit through Holy Saturday. Father said, Christ's face was beaten. When He was taken off the cross, His face was smashed. *My Lord, You bled. My Savior, You were broken: swollen and disfigured.*

What is our faith but love for God?

My daughter sang. Her voice was sweeter than honey, and a woman next to me smiled. After a time, my daughter grew pensive and snuggled against me. "I scared," she said. I asked her why, told her there was nothing to be afraid of, but she insisted staring forward at the crucified Christ beside the iconostasis before the altar. "Eeew, bug," she said, pointing at the nailhead that appeared on the top of Christ's feet. Even a two year old could see the ugliness of death, the terror of crucifixion, the hell that was never intended for us, let alone for our Lord. It was there, right before our eyes, and yet, how often I didn't see it. How often I fail to realize what is truly disgustingly terrifying. To accept my place in sin and darkness is too painful. I would rather deny the reality. Would rather feel better right now, warm my hands with something tangible, fill my belly with something handy. If I never gave over to hope that there was more and engaged a routine of going to the Church where others, stronger, prayed, than it would seem easy enough to deny the Truth all together—I wouldn't have experienced it.

What I have chosen to believe, and do, in this life matters when my time on earth has come to an end. Death seems impossible in the face of Life, as beautiful as the daughter in my arms. It isn't popular to suggest these ugly truths, but then, how bright the reality of God is against them. If we realize the true ugliness of death, then we must realize the light of life and the need for God. Saying instead that death isn't so ugly or something to fear is the ultimate lie and the worst way to pull wool over our eyes, making fuzzy what even a two year old can see and tell.

Christians experience the Passion of Christ if they pick up their cross and bear it. One needn't have holes in the palms of their hands, or a gash in the side. The weight of the world presses into one's flesh and makes real the sacrifice of Love that Christ uniquely calls each one to endure. We are not alone. We are always with our Lord in the trials of this life. We pick up the cross and tremble under the weight of the world, but our vision becomes His own, and we walk forward. To the left, the right, distractions abound, and there is temptation to turn, to listen to the shouts: "Crucify!" —Even when spoken by a mere few very early in the morning, as it was with our Lord. It is heavy, and we are worn, how easy it may be to let go, to let down. The knees buckle with the weight, and it is impossible to carry on. *Too weary, my Lord, I am not You.* Like air, so sweet and gentle, carried as a babe in its mothers arms, helped, protected, a warm kiss gives the necessary life. Moving on, going forth, this is all that can be done, there is no choice, and the voices have grown quiet. All is still and soft, like the humid air before a storm. It is gray. The Passion of Christ stops the world that has always been His.

Thump...thump...thump, His heart beats... to be heard. Too much pain to realize that the blood and water gushing from Him is one's own life. In time, life had seemed one's own, full of choices. At the end, the choices are washed away. There is only the Lord, on the cross. At the burial vigil before Pascha, we hymn the victory of the Lord:

> *When You, the Redeemer of all, were placed in a tomb, all hell's powers quaked in fear. Its bars were broken, its gates were smashed. Its mighty reign was brought to an end, for the dead came forth alive from their tombs, casting off their captivity. Adam was filled with joy. He gratefully cried out to You, O Christ: Glory to Your condescension, O Lover of mankind.*

God's love is not an idea, expression, point of view, or religion. The distractions of life busy us so that we do not often feel the bittersweet fullness of God's love, which is usually more than one can bear. The Pascha of our Lord and Savior Jesus Christ is "Christ is Risen!" and the trampling down of death and illness, of all evil and corruption that numbs us to Love. We don't always feel this, but like the fact of death in this world, is the fact of life in the next.

The body of Christ spans the whole world, and in the power of the faithful, we may close our eyes and listen to the chorus of love that we are too weak to sing in a given moment. We may doubt the reality of Pascha, but we awaken to a bright morning radiant with sunshine and birds chirping in trees beginning to bud. The order of the universe shows us something the heart intuits as faith, despite the distraction of dishes, and breakfast, and a full house. There is natural order and harmony, and the Liturgy of Truth unfolds always, even outside of a church where one's own needy children whimper and distract. Friends' voice the greeting: Christ is Risen! Indeed.... Each life is a vital part of nature, a body that builds the Body and reveals the Spirit from ages to ages, Amen.

EPILOGUE
Holiness and Wholeness in Orthodox Christianity

"Silence in the face of evil is itself evil: God will not hold us guiltless. Not to speak is to speak. Not to act is to act."[201]

We know better—we do better. No room for guilt.

Life is regenerative. As one who was infertile thirteen years before and now has five children, I believe and say: The Giver of Life abides in us, cleanses us from every impurity, and saves our souls.

The effort we make to live for God in our bodies and spirits is what matters most in this life. If we haven't been told what is good and what is not, we can unintentionally harm life. I have written about the risks of vaccination to prevent further harm. The Church has issued a statement declaring the moral responsibility Orthodox Christians have to be vigilant for Life. I have also aimed to show through my personal faith journey how the soul and body are always interacting.

There was a time when I didn't know that fetal stem cells were used in vaccination, or that the ingredients included peanut oil that could sensitize my son to a life-long anaphylactic allergy. There was a time when I wondered if medication for depression might be a way to dull the intensity of life and help ease experiences day to day. For a time, stress and anxiety seemed a natural part of every day. Prayer, coupled with runs outside, helped me manage life. When stress was tight in my gut, I placed my faith in good-intentioned doctors and endured many tests. Throughout my journey towards wellness, prayer has remained a constant. There have been times when praying seemed more natural, and times when prayers were as though far-away bells, chiming in a distant place where my heart longed to be.

In illness, I was close to God. Facing infertility issues, I turned to the Mother of God in a powerful way. Through my prayers to her, and with great desire for new life, wholeness and holiness became clearly grounded in prayer. Prayer has healing effects on a person. Ultimately, it is God, the Master Physician, Who alone reaches into a person and makes well. The journey to God is rarely a linear path, but the road is beautiful because it is true and ends in life.

---

201 Cadwallader, Mark, on Deitrich Bonhoeffer's quote: "Silence in the face of evil is itself evil," http://www.creationmoments.com/content/silence-face-evil-itself-evil, Creation Moments, 2015, web, 17 Oct. 2015.

Re-integration of the human person is the way to holistic wellness, and it occurs through prayer. Fr. Roman Braga says[202] the Lord prays inside one's heart with the genuine, concentrated utterance of "Jesus Christ." When I am running on the treadmill in the basement early in the morning, my body and spirit can enter a methodic trance-like pattern of moving and thinking. My intention is to continue with the Jesus Prayer, but I have found a strange thing sometimes occurs. After saying, "Lord Jesus Christ, have mercy on me, a sinner," I sometimes lose focus on Christ and switch over to counting. I have noticed that the centering effect of having my body move and concentrate continues, and it benefits my body and spirit. However, the experience differs from praying "Jesus Christ" because soon into counting, concerns begin to peak out: what groceries we need, who to text, when to do a million and 20 things.

Truthfully, in the course of prayer, or numeric meditation, as it may be, flooding peace is not the first feeling. Rather, the feeling at first is an uncomfortable wrestling with the aspects of myself that resist submission to God. While a part of me wills to control myself, to hope for a good day and work my body and mind into a state that might allow for this, there is a pull to give in to irritations, to believe that I need this or that, or to flatly deny that God is everywhere present. Other times, I run outside in the morning. In springtime, when I jog, it is a sheer pleasure to feel the breeze against my skin and hear life awakening in the morning. Lake Erie by our home is vast and my face smiles like sunshine spreading through the sky. Such beauty is soft and beyond me, the outside world moves my heart to peace. In the light of early day, it can seem easier to praise God by prayer in my spirit and body. Even in times when prayer is easier and earthly goodness obvious, the experience of Peace in Christ is something independent of any and every earthly care. There is nothing that can break or infect salvation: nothing. I am well, in a dark basement, or free among the morning's song. In prayer that envelops my children, husband, job, health, and the world itself, my will in Christ is Peace. Prayer humbles me.

I have heard it said that death is the "equalizer;" it levels us all to dust. It doesn't get more humbling than that. As Fr. Thomas Hopko says, we are to make death to die so that life can live, but death has been naturalized. We don't realize it as an enemy. If we don't see death for what it is, we remain stuck in false confidence. Our confidence in ourselves steals our attention from our Savior.

In today's western health care system, we tend to place our confidence not directly in ourselves but in pharmaceuticals that can free us from having to suffer and convince us that death hasn't a sting. We place confidence in vaccines to keep us free of disease, though there are a myriad of potential physical and spiritual harms that result from injecting aborted fetal stem cells with trace amounts of foreign human DNA and harmful adjuvants and preservatives into human persons. This book has led me on a journey to

---

202 Metropulos, Fr. Chris, "Finding God in Prayer: an interview with Fr. Roman Braga," http://myocn.net/finding-god-in-prayer/, Orthodox Christian Network, 28 May 2015, web, 17 Oct. 2015.

understanding vaccination and has landed me on a realization that our body and soul is one: personhood is beautiful, holy, a gift worthy of all our protection and nurturing.

My journey into vaccine awareness began with a quest to understand the effects on the body, and it continues on with appreciation of the synergism between a person's body and spirit. I have presented others' arguments that vaccines cause diseases through viral shedding and over-taxing immune systems with harmful ingredients. I have also presented their claims that vaccines cause brain damage, including autism. Mandating vaccination violates our right to medical freedom and our own bodies, placing lives in the hands of the state. History has shown the ill effects of relinquishing our bodies and souls to governing powers, just look at Nazi Germany in the 1940s. To all of this, I wish to conclude by beseeching others to realize the violation of our souls when we harm innocent children and abort babies in the name of medical science. I hold hope that many others also care deeply about honoring God, and so we must reject bills that could enslave us by objecting before they are passed. We must refuse to follow doctors that could scare us into vaccination, and become aware and active in our families and local communities.

Vaccines do not warrant our trust, and they never have. Studies are skewed, and there is an alternative agenda. For example, "The results of the latest study about vaccines and autism are in, and they're not surprising[203]," Eric March reports that vaccines do not cause autism. In the article, SafeMinds, supposedly an anti-vaccine group, funded and conducted a study over more than ten years, beginning in 2003 to 2013. The article begins: "Here's the thing about science. It has a mind of its own. And sometimes, it won't do what you want it to do." March continues, "It's one thing to spend money on honest scientific inquiry and let the chips fall where they may. But once the inquiry has been made, it's important to respect the facts." And with the following, he delivers the expected bottom line: "Everyone is entitled to their own opinion, but no one is entitled to their own science." Facts are subjectively read and interpreted by human subjects, and building the immune system strong against disease is a complex process explained variously. In response to the above research, VaxTruth investigates[204] by reading the study with critical attention to the research itself. It was found that the number of macaque participants, timeframe of the vaccinations, and the results on the participants' brains as a whole are skewed. Countless parents have observed brain damage in their children after vaccination. March's argument is very acceptable in our western culture to many people, but as more chronic conditions develop in more children, parents wonder if there are other ways to understand wellness—and to explain what is harming our children.

---

203 March, Eric, "The results of the latest study about vaccines and autism are in, and they're not surprising," http://upworthy.com/the-results-of-the-latest-study-about-vaccines-and-autism-are-in-and-theyre-not-surprising?g=2&c=ufb1, Upworthy, 06 Oct. 2015, web, 06 Oct. 2015.
204 Marcella, "Newest Macaque Study on Vaccines and Autism is Bunk," http://vaxtruth.org/2015/10/macaquebunk/, VaxTruth, 04 Oct. 2015, web, 06 Oct. 2015.

In his recent speech on the corruption surrounding the CDC's vaccine division, Robert F. Kennedy, Jr. commented on the socio-political ramifications of our current system of vaccination.[205] He stands pro-choice concerning vaccines, warning the public against mandatory vaccination, because the research overwhelmingly illustrates current vaccines are not safe and are being pushed for financial reasons. Additionally, the CDC is not serving as a regulatory agency with integrity and credibility. He argues that government officials ought to be focusing on restoring integrity to the CDC.

> Because the CDC is a very troubled agency, and it's not just me saying this. There have been four separate, scathing, federal studies by the United States Congress: a three-year study by Congressman Burton, a follow-up study by Senator Coburn's committee, another study by the inspector general of the Department of Health and Human Services (HHS) in 2008, and a study last year by the Office of Research Integrity of HHS. All of those studies paint the CDC as an absolute cesspool of corruption, as an agency that has fallen under the spell of this trillion-dollar Big Pharma industry. Instead of serving its primary mission, which is to protect public health, its mission now, according to these federal studies, is to serve the mercantile interests of the vaccine industry.

Kennedy claims that there are two areas of corruption in the CDC's vaccine division. The first is the division choosing which vaccines to add to the schedule. Vaccines are made, and the federal government orders people to buy them. "There's no advertising, there's no market, the patents never expire, and [they] can't be sued. So no matter how badly [they] make that product, no matter how many defects it has in it, nobody can ever hold [them] accountable." In 2008, the Inspector General of the HHS report said that "virtually all of the members of those committees have financial entanglements with the vaccine companies." He provided an illustration with Dr. Paul Offit, who sat on a committee to ensure that the rotavirus vaccine be added to the schedule, and who gained $40 million for himself in producing a rotavirus vaccine and selling the patent six years later. Instead of doctors and scientists gathering to discuss vaccines during committee hearings, there are "a bunch of Wall Street analysts in suits. Moreover, as soon as that decision is made, they run out of the room and get on their cell phones and you can watch that stock price spike. So these are financial decisions that are being driven by a trillion-dollar industry and we need to restore the integrity of that agency."

The second area of corruption is the scientists deciding the safety and efficacy of vaccines, the immunology safety division of the CDC:

> But what we now know, from looking at the science and the phony epidemiological studies that they produce, is that this division is extremely corrupt. A senior scientist at the CDC, a 17-year veteran, Dr. William Thompson,

205 Kennedy Jr., "Unchecked Power | Informed Choice," http://pathwaystofamilywellness.org/Informed-Choice/unchecked-power.html, Pathways to Family Wellness, issue #47, 2015, web, 17 Oct. 2015.

who is the lead author on the most important of those studies, has now invoked, as of August, federal whistleblower protection, and has hired Morgan Verkamp, one of the leading whistleblower attorneys in our country. [He] has said publicly that the CDC scientists in that division have been required by their bosses for at least a decade to lie, to manipulate, to massage data, and to bury data that connect neurological disorders including autism to thimerosal exposure and to vaccines. And he has turned over tens of thousands of pages of documents to Congress and he wants to be subpoenaed and to testify so that the American press will finally have to begin covering something that we have known about for a decade. So here is the problem: All of the checks and balances in our society that normally would protect children from a rapacious industry have been neutralized.

The root causes of some children's health conditions are vaccines. I read a very sad story of a father who had spent his life fighting against health care norms in order to help his daughter become more well. It was a futile situation from the beginning, as he hadn't known how to help his daughter with many health problems, though he was adamant that she should not be given medications. It began when his small daughter was vaccinated. She developed a "strange" reaction of arthritis in childhood. It became severe and she was in a wheelchair. She continued to be ill, and the father fought doctors with the wish not to medicate his daughter because of the medications' heinous side effects. After researching the benefit of fasting, he led his daughter to a facility where they helped her become more well through more naturalistic approaches, including fasting. The child became a young woman, married, and had two children. The family increasingly fell into disarray, and even used illicit drugs for a time. The woman's condition deteriorated and she ended up in a hospital. The father was still involved and insisted that she not be treated with strong medications, but she was anyways. The father was deeply troubled to continue learning how health care providers used medication, despite the ill effects on his daughter. In the end, the daughter was placed in a nursing home and killed through medication that triggered a fatal heart condition. There was no apology, and the father was left with much pain and no answers.

In *Becoming Whole: Building Natural Immunity in the Body and Soul* the experiences we have in our bodies, observations of our children, and prayers we engage with our very lives foster faith, which enlivens holiness. Because a human being is body and spirit, becoming holy and becoming whole is related, and this is my main argument throughout this book. My message is more than an argument. It is a confession that the Giver of Life is infinitely merciful and good, and He gives us Life, without our earning it.

Bantering back-and-forth with my husband in the kitchen as the small girls noisily played and the boys argued over a game, I locked his eyes and confessed that we didn't deserve the life God had given us. It was my admittance to myself that it would be impossible for God to grant us another child, even though it seemed in my heart that there was yet to be one. When I realized that I was pregnant, the overwhelming feeling that God gives what we do not deserve, according to His purposes, overcame me. I was quiet that early morning, absorbing the mercy of the Lord against the silence of the January pre-dawn sky. The goodness of God goes against the pronouncement that Dr. Andrew Wakefield recently made: If we continue vaccinations as planned, no one will be left. The threat against the sanctity of life cannot win out over the mercy of the Lord. That is my final and triumphant point.

Life is hard. We are meant to work, to make effort, and to rest in the next life, as Fr. Hopko said as he was dying. While there are times when we cannot do this on our own, many other times we can, if we think that we have to. A person is never alone. God helps us in all things. He can and does help us through medications, but we have lost touch with the necessity of personal responsibility for wellness through food and lifestyle. All can heal. All can become more well. The soul can be saved—with effort and good works that allow God's grace and mercy to indeed save us.

The physical and emotional struggles we face in this life can lead us into despair. I believe and have experienced prayer as the chief remedy for sadness. I am inspired by Orthodoxy where Saints and their icons continue to show us the light of Jesus Christ in this world. For a few years now, an icon of the Mother of God in Taylor, PA has been streaming myrrh. Since the icon began to stream myrrh, Fr. Mark Leasure promised God that he would serve a Moleben service every Wednesday until the second coming of Christ. He has. People have been healed. Health care professionals, not all Christian, have even come to have their hands anointed with the myrrh. Four years before, there were fewer than 50 congregants at the Moleben service. Now, there are over one-thousand who travel, some far distances, to St. George Carpatho-Russian Orthodox Church for the experience. In one instance, a woman was suffering terminal brain cancer. From the service, she anointed herself with a cotton ball drenched in the myrrh from the icon, and she slept with the myrrh under her pillow for a time. One morning she awoke to a mass on her pillow and a substance flowing from her nose. After going to the hospital and following tests, it was determined that the tumor had expelled itself from her body and she was healed. In another situation, a gentleman had passed out while in service. The icon of the Mother of God was held above him, the myrrh falling upon him. The gentleman inhaled deeply and awoke, singing, "Most Holy Theotokos, save us."

On the Feast of the Transfiguration at The Monastery of the Transfiguration in P.A., I saw this icon, inhaled the scent of heaven, like roses but better, and longed to take some home. When someone rubbed the myrrh over my baby's hair, I wept with joy. Similar to myrrh-streaming icons, with their scent of heaven, we are to be icons of Christ. As 2 Corinthians 14-15 says: "Now thanks be to God who always leads us in triumph in Christ, and through us diffuses the fragrance of His knowledge in every place. For we are to God the fragrance of Christ among those who are being saved and among those who are perishing."

In the Orthodox Church, the Faith is alive through the sensate experiences of her people. The feelings in the heart, the scents, sights, sounds, these are all ways of knowing God, and they are no less than understanding the history and theology of the Faith. We are created to know God through the faculties of our being. When we catch a glimpse of God's love and intuit that this love is for us, then we feel amazing tenderness. We love God, and this love can spill out of me for others. Against God's love, my sins are clear, and I regret them. My priest commented during a service for Holy Week that he has yet to weep for his sins, despite the rich lamentations in the hymnology of the Church throughout Lent, and especially Holy Week. In fact, my priest said, to be able to weep for one's sins is understood as a spiritual gift in the Church.

Life becomes a prayer through choices one makes continually through a day. All of life's circumstances are opportunities by which life may become prayer, if one wills to repent from sin and seek God. St. Seraphim of Sarov says that the difference between a saint and a sinner is one's resolve not to sin. Fr. Lawrence Farley says,

> [S]alvation consists in giving one's life, heart, and soul to God, living and dying for Him down to one's last breath and one's last drop of blood. The issue is: may we give such loyalty, allegiance, love, and commitment to Jesus of Nazareth, or not? If He is not truly God, then giving Him such allegiance would be idolatry. No one sensibly would live and die so totally for a mere celebrity. [But, it is for one's] salvation that we bow the knee in love to Him, even now before the final end, and confess that the road to His city runs through our heart.[206]

My priest commented on the parable we read at Pascha about the one who comes to Christ at the eleventh hour. Even though it is "last minute," the choice is made for God, and he has time in this life to live for God. In another similar parable, workers toil all day and receive pay the same as those who work but one hour. The message is clear that even if one's life is not spent entirely in serving God, if a portion of life is, we will be saved. We think we'll get to God later, my priest said, but we do not know when the end will be.

God's love is not reserved for a few but is freely given to everyone. The experience of God's love is transformational and healing. I spoke with a woman whose nephew had been a neo-Nazi. He was heavily tattooed with swastikas and various harsh signs of intolerance. After a time, he began to turn away from a life of hate but resisted God with feelings of unworthiness. He asked, "Does God hate me? Look at me," he said, staring down at his hands where tattooed knuckles were in fists. He wondered how God could possibly forgive him. His aunt said to simply ask God to forgive him. This young man was

---

206 Farley, Fr. Lawrence, "The Fathers of Nicea. Why Should I Care?" St. Nicholas Orthodox Church, Mentor, OH, parish bulletin, 24 May 2015.

cleaning a gun a short time later when it went off and a bullet shot into his forehead. Family came to say goodbye as he survived for a number of days, cared for with complete tenderness and compassion in the hands of nurses and medical staff that were various races and orientations. Ironically, this young man had been blinded by his own hands to all the differences that had led him from Love in his lifetime. In the end, he was granted a peaceful death, and essentially, he was embraced by humanity—by what it means to be made in the image and likeness of Christ Himself.

It was early spring and my husband and older children spent the day traveling to a relative's. My mother and father came for lunch with the girls and me. The relationship with my parents has always been open and loving. As I grow older, I appreciate their kindness and their way of life that includes daily walks down the street I grew up on to Lake Erie. My mother and father sat in my living room as we shared an afternoon cup of coffee. The toddler danced with music she found on my cell phone, and the baby laughed on the floor, fists in her eager mouth. The living room was bright from sunshine on snow outside the windows. Thirty-six years earlier, my grandmother told my mom to love me, that was all that she needed to worry about. Looking at my mother and feeling all that she is to me after these 36 years, I understood Love. It was an experience of complete goodness that drew me to give all I could.

Sometimes the horrors of an evil world seem far away and we'd rather not imagine them. Even death seems like a distant reality, until one or one's loved one personally suffers. Yet, to pray for the world means to care for the world, and realizing that others suffer persecution and martyrdom is important. Salvation is a great gift, and we all need it, but sometimes in a comfortable situation it seems that one doesn't need God. My parents and I talked about the attacks of ISIS on Orthodox Christians in the Middle East, the beheadings of 21 Coptic Christians, and the mutilation of children and women professing faith in Christ. Such evil has roots in Satan's active delusion of one's will: "A lie is a delusion of the mind, while evil is a delusion of the will. The sign by which one is distinguished from the other is the judgement of God Himself [...] Truth is that which leads a man to will for good. But whatever contradicts this is entirely false, entirely evil."[207] Even though we couldn't feel it in my living room that sun-drenched winter's day, evil roamed this world.

No matter what horrors we might have to experience, God is with us and reveals Himself in unexpected times and ways. St. Silouan the Athonite says, "Don't be troubled if you don't feel the love of God in yourself, but think about the Lord, that He is merciful, and guard yourself from sins, and the grace of God will teach you."[208] My father

207 Cabasilas, St. Nicholas, *Three-hundred Sayings of the Ascetics of the Orthodox Church*, http://orthodox.cn/patristics/300sayings_en.htm, Ven. Serapion Kozheozersky, ed., Moscow, Orthodox Missionary Society, 2011, web, 01 June 2015.
208 Athonite, St. Silouan the, "Writings, IX. 16," http://orthodox.cn/patristics/300sayings_en.htm, *Three-hundred Sayings of the Ascetics of the Orthodox Church*, Ven. Serapion Kozheozersky, ed., Moscow, Orthodox Missionary Society, 2011, web, 01 June 2015.

commented on the Lord's Prayer, "Your will be done, on earth as it is in heaven," saying that he thought it was given to us because the Lord knew its relevance for all ages.

The Church is the Mother that teaches us Love. Holy Orthodoxy preserves Christ's tradition of loving us, and calling us to love one another. Sadly, our nation's disjointed Christianity's weaken our unity in Jesus Christ. Holy Orthodoxy is the rich, deep Faith that was established from the time of Christ, and our nation would stand stronger united together in the Faith. Together, our prayers would have that much more power against the evil one who is actively troubling the world. Christians must preserve the sanctity of life and draw together in common faith in order to do so with more effect in this broken world.

The boys returned home after six that evening and darted out of the car. My husband grabbed hats, gloves, and a football for the kids as I re-bundled the babies to satisfy Daddy that they truly were not cold. Spring was in the foreseeable distance, and though we walked along mounds of icy-snow, it was turning brown and slushy. In the moment, I chose to believe in the miracle of the world's rebirth, marveling that God sustained life through the ages. After a dinner of fried potatoes, asparagus, and tuna cakes, I cuddled with the boys.

We are like the only Orthodox, they said. *Why you care so much about church*, they asked. I was quiet and heavy with the desire to make my faith their own. I longed for the Faith to be more visibly expressed in their lives, for neighbors and family to demonstrate an active love for God. I thought of a story from a friend who traveled to Greece during Great Lent where even in the restaurants fish entrees indicated to patrons that the time was touched by a cycle of faith. "Let us fast like children," we hymned at church. How true it is that children are naturally less concerned with the satisfactions of the flesh because there is a wide world in which they long to explore. Their joy is not dependent on cake, even though they surely enjoy it. They laugh, wrestle, and fully engage with life, so long as they are provided the space to do so. The boys fell asleep while a dread fear awoke in my mind. I wondered how I could possibly show them what it is that I believe: that God is true, that nothing matters so much as living for Him. I worried that in our saturated culture, they would not experience an Orthodox cycle of faith. How would a definite, fighting love for God awaken in my children? It would require an inner fight against sin that separates each of us from God, but only love of the Lord would inspire the effort towards holiness. They had to feel my love, God's love, and know it deep inside their souls.

That night, I slipped notes into their lunch-boxes saying that God was sitting next to them, encouraging them to talk to Him. A bit cheesy but from the heart. Would my faith influence theirs? Did Christ's light of joy shine, despite my limitations? I despaired that I could not make faith real enough for them that it was ultimately up to each one's own body and spirit to experience prayer and perceive Him. I would give them anything, but it was so hard to have to give them nothing—only my prayers. My husband was strong and silent, and I cuddled against his back as he slept. There was no one to whom I could turn but the Lord Himself. Prayer flowed through me in tender silence.

On the day of resurrection, will God know me? Will I know God?

To know Him is to be known by Him.

The lives of Sts. Seraphim and Herman show how powerful life can be when a person uses the body, whether broken or whole, in ways pleasing to God. I have heard, "What the soul is in the body, Christians are in the world."[209] The body may be weak, as was St. Seraphim of Sarov's after robbers beat him almost to death and he lived the rest of his days with a crippled back. My priest said that St. Seraphim walked through the forest in the night and glowed because there was so much God in him that it had to find its way out. The body may be strong, as was St. Herman of Alaska's. He was a strong man who helped the natives in Alaska. He showed them how to build, cook, garden, and pray. He walked barefooted through the Alaskan forest in the winter carrying tree trunks on his back. When asked how he could manage as a small man, he said that it was God in him Who made him so strong.

Though each person has her own unique strengths and ailments, all people benefit from realizing that the body and spirit are in symbiosis. Everything done in the body matters—for the good of the spirit. As St. Seraphim says, acquire a peaceful spirit and a thousand others will be saved. A peaceful spirit is possible on one's deathbed, but there is less time and less energy to move through the forest of life and allow God's uncreated light to shine through one's own body, as it did for St. Seraphim.

My friend Dn. Stephen Muse is a psychotherapist interested in the body and spirit relationship. He has worked with traumatized persons whose bodies re-experienced the physical pain from their early childhood dissociated experience as they began to recover. He traveled to India and met an 85-year-old nun named Ammachi Susan. She had not eaten food in 60 years and lived off Eucharist and water, sometimes a little juice. A CT scan showed her intestine like a straight line, which didn't function. He said, "Hers is the only case of Orthodox (albeit Malankaran) with stigmata[210] I have ever heard of." She has had this since age 13. He wonders about the relationship between Ammachi Susan's early pain in her family and her later identification with the physical agony of Jesus. He tells of a colleague whose patient had a wound open on her throat when she began to emotionally re-experience the trauma she went through as a child being choked with a rope around her neck.

---

209 "From a Letter to Diognetus: The Christian in the World,"
http://www.vatican.va/spirit/documents/spirit_20010522_diogneto_en.html, 22 May 2001, web, 01 Oct. 2015.
210 In Christian tradition, marks on the body that correspond to the Crucifixion.

Such stories, and our own lives, reveal that our bodies and spirits interact in amazing ways. The intricacies of the body and spirit are unfathomable. The meaning of our lives is beyond any medical and spiritual tradition. One should not expect to be well, but one can pray for the gift of health in order to be more useful for God's purposes. Sometimes one is most useful in illness. God alone realizes the full picture of one's life. The task at hand is to pray with one's very life. If one realizes the symbiosis of the body and spirit, then one perceives the Body of Christ, which is the Church. All Truth is found in God, and Wisdom is as near as one is close to God.

Saving souls, those I love and even my own, is not up to me. It is up to God. He asks me to pray to Him, holding all others in my heart as I do so. My baptism into Christ wed my heart, hands, mind, and feet to God. The best I can do is use my body, mind, spirit, heart—all of myself—to the glory of God. Each one is created to know God in a personal, real way. My heart fears, because I long for Him so little. Most of my striving is for little faith in ways of life that fit within my limited understanding. I believe, according to the Faith, that I will stand before the dread judgment seat of Christ. His uncreated light—a mystery of Love—will illumine every detail of my life. I shudder. *God, my God, Who are You?* Inside me a voice ventures, *Are you concerned with Truth?*

May the Saints pray for us here on earth struggling to serve God. St. Xenia was known as a fool for Christ. May her prayers help and guide those who read this work, as speaking against vaccination in the face of widespread cultural ignorance makes one seem "foolish." May St. Theophan the Recluse pray for us sinners as we feel the pain of realizing vaccination is harmful and the pain of trying to tell others who are not ready to listen. St. Theophan says, "The organ of speech is the only bodily organ that is intended to serve the soul." May we realize that the body and the soul is wed, and that what we do in the body is always also spiritual. Since the beginning of this book, I have thought that if one realizes the body and soul are in synergistic relationship, then one perceives the Body of Christ, which is the Church. May it be so.

How does one know the Truth?
Seek Love, Who is God.
How does one seek God?
Obey the spirit of Love, which is the law.
What are acts of love?

Care of family,
Friends,
And all others as one's self.

ABOUT THE AUTHOR

Lea is married to Dimitri and they live in Ohio with their five children. They attend St. Nicholas Orthodox Church where they were baptized 13 years ago. They believe in the sanctity of life and aim to honor the Life Giver, despite the struggle that is common in today's daily life. It is imperative that Christians recognize that the body and soul is one. Lea says, "It matters what we do in our bodies. As those who profess faith in the Giver of Life, there is no valid argument for using vaccines. They are not good for our health, and they are produced using fetal stem cells."

Lea and Dima enjoy spending time in nature with their family: from hikes in the Upper Peninsula, MI, on summer camping trips, to national parks throughout Ohio, they find connection and release in nature.

Lea holds a PhD in English and an MFA in Creative Writing. She has a memoir on becoming a multicultural family and converting to the Orthodox Church from Protestantism: *Finding Love, Family, and God: Living the Orthodox Christian Tradition* (2016).

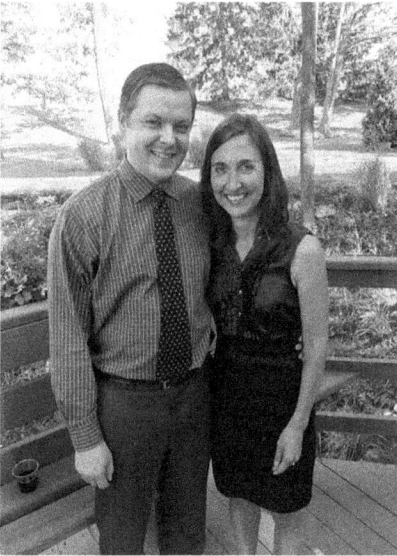

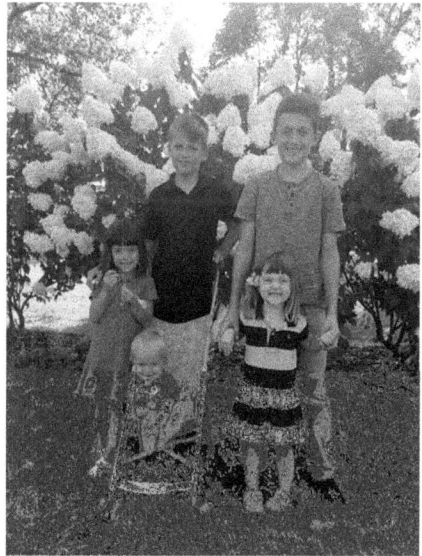

www.ingramcontent.com/pod-product-compliance
Lightning Source LLC
Chambersburg PA
CBHW072013290326
41934CB00007BA/1080